The OIE Global Conference on Aquatic Animal Health

••••••••••••••••••

Developments in Biologicals

Vol.129

This series"Developments in Biologicals" begins vith vol.102 and is the continuation of IABS symposia series "Progress in Immunobiological Standardization", Vol 1-5, "Immunobiological Standardization", Vols 1-22 and "Developments in Biological Standardization", Vols 23-101.

Organized and published by the International Association for Biologicals (IABS)

KARGER

Basel . Freiburg . Paris . London . New York
Bangalore . Bangkok . Singapore . Tokyo . Sydney

The OIE Global Conference on Aquatic Animal Health

Bergen, Norway
9-12 October 2006

Volume editors *Betty Dodet*
International Association for Biologicals (IABS)
DBS

In collaboration with the Scientific and Technical Department of the OIE

Technical editor *Marissa Vicari*

Proceedings of a global conference organised by the
World Organisation for Animal Health – OIE

27 figures and 14 tables, 2007

KARGER

Basel . Freiburg . Paris . London . New York
Bangalore . Bangkok . Singapore . Tokyo . Sydney

Developments in Biologicals

Library of Congress Cataloging-in-Publication Data

OIE Global Conference on Aquatic Animal Health (2006 : Bergen, Norway)
The OIE Global Conference on Aquatic Animal Health, Bergen, Norway, 9-12 October 2006 / volume editors, Betty Dodet ; in collaboration with the Scientific and Technical Department of the OIE ; technical editor, Marissa Vicari.
p. cm. -- (Developments in biologicals ; v. 129)
Includes bibliographical references.
ISBN 978-3-8055-8344-2 (soft cover : alk. paper)
1. Aquatic animals--Health--Congresses. I. Dodet, Betty. II. International Office of Epizootics III. Title.
SF997.5.A65O34 2007
636.089--dc22

2007038029

Bibliographic Indices. This publication is listed in bibliographic services, including Current Contents® and Index Medicus.

Drug dosage. The authors and the publisher have exerted every effort to ensure that drug selection and dosage set forth in this text are in accord with current recommendations and practice at the time of publication. However, in view of ongoing research, changes in government regulations, and the constant flow of information relating to drug therapy and drug reactions, the reader is urged to check the package insert for each drug for any change in indications and dosage and for added warnings and precautions. This is particularly important when the recommended agent is a new and/or infrequently employed drug.

Worldwide distribution by S. Karger AG, Basel (Switzerland).
Printed in France by IML, Saint-Matin-en-haut (France).
ISBN 978-3-8055-8344-2

The scientific integrity of the articles contained in this volume is the sole responsibility of the authors.

Steering Committee

K. Bar-Yaacov (Chief Veterinary Officer Norway)
K. Thorud (Senior advisor, Ministry of Fisheries and Coastal Affairs)
J.-L. Angot (OIE)
D. Wilson (OIE)
C. Bruschke (OIE)

Scientific Committee

E.-M. Bernoth (President of the Aquatic Animal Health Standards Commission)
B. Hill (Vice-President of the Aquatic Animal Health Standards Commission)
T. Håstein (National Veterinary Institute)
M. Binde (Norwegian Food Safety Authority)
F. Berthe (Atlantic Veterinary College, University of Prince Edward Island)
D.V. Lightner (University of Arizona, USA)

Organisation of the Scientific Programme

Session I	Introduction
Session II	Cooperation among Stakeholders in Aquatic Animal Disease Management
Session III	Infrastructure for Disease Surveillance and Emergency Response
Session IV	Communication and Networking
Session V	Education and Training Needs in Aquatic Animal Health
Session VI	Aquatic Animal Welfare
Session VII	Conference Recommendations and the Way Forward

Acknowledgements

The OIE is grateful for the very valuable support of the Norwegian Ministry of Fisheries and Coastal Affairs, the Norwegian Food Safety Authority, the National Veterinary Institute and the Institute of Marine Research of Norway. The OIE also acknowledges the support of Travel Planners of Scandinavia Ltd.

Contents

Preface

For over forty years the remit of the World Organisation for Animal Health (OIE) has included aquatic animals. The OIE would like to reinforce the commitment of its Member Countries to their obligations regarding disease notification and implementation of OIE standards in line with the SPS Agreement of the World Trade Organization. Furthermore the International Committee of the OIE, at the 72nd General Session, endorsed a set of recommendations to improve cooperation between veterinary and fisheries authorities on aquatic animal health matters in order to facilitate the implementation of the international obligations of Member Countries.

Among the specific recommendations are that OIE " reinforce to Delegates their responsibility to the OIE for terrestrial as well as aquatic animals "; " request Member Countries to clarify the roles and responsibilities for aquatic animal health assigned to veterinary and other authorities in their country "; and " provide opportunities to assist cooperation between veterinary and other authorities responsible for aquatic animal health in Member Countries ..."; and " request their Veterinary Services to improve the communication and cooperation with fishery authorities, especially regarding disease reporting and disease emergency responses ".

This OIE Global Conference on Aquatic Animal Health will provide an opportunity to assist the OIE and its Member Countries in exchanging the latest information on developing a science-based approach to the management of aquatic animal health and welfare, and to present the valuable experience gained in the past few years. The presentations and discussions will assist in the evaluation and improvement of the current standards and guidelines for better control of infectious aquatic animal health and countries' capabilities to prepare for and respond to aquatic animal disease emergencies, as well as better defining roles and responsibilities.

Thanks to the hospitality of the Government of Norway and our Norwegian colleagues, it is expected that all Member Countries will benefit from this International Conference. I welcome all of you to the OIE Global Conference on Aquatic Animal Health.

Dr. Bernard Vallat
OIE Director General

Dodet B, the OIE Scientific & Technical Department (eds): The OIE Global Conference on Aquatic Animal Health. Dev Biol (Basel). Basel, Karger, 2007, vol 129, p 1.

Session I

Introduction

Dodet B, the OIE Scientific & Technical Department (eds): The OIE Global Conference on Aquatic Animal Health. Dev Biol (Basel). Basel, Karger, 2007, vol 129, pp 3-4.

Opening Remarks

We are all gathered here in Bergen these two days to discuss some very central themes for those who work in the field of aquatic animal health and welfare and hopefully for those who are considering how to become more involved in the future.

The objectives of the conference are to help build a framework for improved involvement and cooperation between the Authorities (Veterinary and Fish Health, Fisheries and Environment), the scientific community and the private sector on aquatic animal health and welfare; help clarify the roles and responsibilities of all stakeholders in the process of early disease detection, rapid response and reporting; help increase aquatic animal health emergency response capabilities; exchange information on emerging diseases and animal welfare issues and help develop a science based approach to the management of aquatic animal health and welfare.

We have prepared a programme that we hope may contribute to these objectives and we intend to finalise the Conference with some recommendations on the way forward. The programme includes sessions on cooperation among stakeholders in aquatic animal disease management, infrastructure for disease surveillance and emergency response, communication and networking, education and training needs and finally a separate session on aquatic animal welfare.

Aquaculture is one of the fastest growing industries globally and, according to the latest statistics, now provides over 40% of all fisheries production. Production volume from aquaculture will surpass that of traditional fisheries in a few years and is fast becoming one of our main sources of animal protein globally. New species and methodologies contribute to the fact that new emerging diseases are increasingly discovered within this field and animal welfare issues are really just in the starting blocks.

Why not copy all that has already been done within terrestrial disease and welfare management? There are many similarities, but there are also many essential differences. The aquaculture industry has very quickly become big business with owner structures that in some countries are more reminiscent of the oil industry conglomerates rather than of traditional farming structures. Management in many countries started where the fish were, in other words in the fisheries. Veterinary Authorities in many countries have not been knowledgeable enough and therefore have not tried to play a role. It is important that they now latch on to make a strong and durable partnership, rather than competing against each other. Traditional veterinary training has not focused on aquatic physiology or the aquatic environment, which we all know is very different from land and air, while we still believe that basic pathology and medicine are also important assets to utilise. Future managers need to have a good mix of veterinary, biological and environmental competences.

Research in many countries is focusing more and more on better production and better quality, but we need more knowledge concerning new and possibly devastating diseases, not to mention future animal welfare issues. If basic research isn't given priority it is very difficult to give science based advice when a crisis arises.

Aquatic animals have been part of the OIE remit for almost fifty years. Through this conference and a future Scientific Review we hope to help the Member Countries focus on the central issues. We need to make sure that we all recognise our separate roles and responsibilities and are prepared to work together for the future.

Dr. Keren Bar-Yaacov
Chief Veterinary Officer

Dodet B, the OIE Scientific & Technical Department (eds): The OIE Global Conference on Aquatic Animal Health. Dev Biol (Basel). Basel, Karger, 2007, vol 129, pp 5-10.

Setting the Scene for the OIE Global Conference on Aquatic Animal Health

E.-M. Bernoth

President, OIE Aquatic Animal Health Standards Commission, Office of the Chief Veterinary Officer, Australian Government Department of Agriculture, Fisheries and Forestry, Canberra, Australia

Key words: OIE, Fish Diseases Commission, Nouméa Recommendations, Asia

INTRODUCTION

The OIE (World Organisation for Animal Health) is an intergovernmental organisation, created in 1924, currently with 167 Member Countries. Its main objectives consist of the following: to ensure transparency in the global animal disease situation; to collect, analyse and disseminate veterinary scientific information; to provide expertise and encourage international solidarity in the control of animal diseases; within its mandate under the WTO SPS Agreement[1] , to safeguard world trade by publishing health standards for international trade in animals and animal products; to improve the legal framework and resources of national Veterinary Services; and to provide a better guarantee for the safety of food of animal origin and to promote animal welfare through a science-based approach.

The OIE's scope has covered aquatic animals for almost fifty years, yet national Delegates of many OIE Member Countries do not seem to fully acknowledge their resulting responsibilities, nor do they use their power to influence the setting of aquatic animal health standards through the OIE as fully as they might. This is of particular concern in the Asian region, where over 80% of the value and over 90% of the volume of aquaculture produce originates [1].

1 World Trade Organization Agreement on the Application of Sanitary and Phytosanitary Measures

The Nouméa Conference

In early 2002, the then OIE Fish Diseases Commission (renamed in 2003 to Aquatic Animal Health Standards Commission; in brief, Aquatic Animals Commission) suggested to the OIE that aquatic animal health should be a "Technical item" at the 23rd Conference of the OIE Regional Commission for Asia, the Far East and Oceania, which was to take place in Nouméa, New Caledonia, in November 2003. The OIE's acceptance of this proposal demonstrates the importance the OIE places on aquatic animal health.

In preparation, a questionnaire was circulated to OIE Member Countries in the region, asking for information regarding the following points: aquaculture and aquatic animal health services; responsible authority; disease reporting; and cooperation with the OIE.

The Technical Item presentation at the "Nouméa Conference" incorporated the responses to the questionnaire. It also drew upon findings of the Aquatic Animals Commission and the Asia Regional Advisory Group on Aquatic Animal Health (established under the Network of Aquaculture Centres in Asia-Pacific, NACA).

The Key Findings Pertaining to the Situation in Asia

Aquaculture and aquatic animal health services

Aquaculture has been growing rapidly in many countries in the region and is predicted to continue to grow in all OIE Member Countries, but there has not been a matching expansion of a supporting aquatic animal health infrastructure, and the aquatic animal sector in the region is currently not as well provided with diagnostic and professional health services as the livestock sector.

OIE Member Countries see an increasing role for health professionals (veterinarians and others) in their country.

Responsible authority

In some OIE Member Countries, fisheries authorities have either the sole responsibility for aquatic animal health or share it with the Veterinary Services. In these countries, fisheries authorities would take the lead in mounting an emergency response to an aquatic animal disease outbreak, and the Veterinary Services are usually well experienced in managing terrestrial animal emergency disease outbreaks, but there is infrequent contact between the two.

Disease reporting

Most OIE Member Countries regularly provide aquatic animal disease reports, but there are numerous reporting errors such as the use of inappropriate symbols; inconsistency between the information provided to the OIE's Regional Office and that provided to the OIE Central Bureau; and not reporting new disease occurrences that would be of major epidemiological significance to other countries in the region.

Cooperation with the OIE

In many OIE Member Countries, draft texts for the OIE *Aquatic Animal Health Code* and the OIE *Manual of Diagnostic Tests for Aquatic Animals* reach aquatic animal health experts either too late or not at all, resulting in few official comments. This means that OIE Member Countries do not sufficiently use the opportunity to influence the setting of international standards that underpin international trade.

The OIE continues to engage in regional aquatic animal health initiatives, together with the Food and Agriculture Organization of the United Nations (FAO) and NACA, but enhanced involvement of both veterinary and fisheries authorities within Member Countries is required to achieve the desired outcomes in areas such as improving OIE Member Countries' knowledge of OIE standard-setting activities in the field of aquatic animal health and the transparency of epidemiological reporting.

The "Nouméa Recommendations"

Based on this Technical Item [2], the OIE Regional Commission for Asia, the Far East and Oceania adopted a number of recommendations (the "Nouméa Recommendations") that were subsequently endorsed by the International Committee of the OIE at the 72nd General Session in May 2004 [3], acknowledging that while the recommendations were based on the situation in Asia, they were globally applicable. The recommendations are shown in full in Figure 1.

72 GS/FR – PARIS, May 2004
23RD CONFERENCE OF THE OIE REGIONAL COMMISSION FOR ASIA, THE FAR EAST AND OCEANIA
Nouméa (New Caledonia), 25-28 November 2003

Recommendation No. 2
Update on developments in aquatic animal diseases

CONSIDERING THAT

Aquaculture has been growing rapidly in many countries in the region and is predicted to continue to grow in all Member Countries,

There has not been a matching expansion of a supporting aquatic animal health infrastructure, and the aquatic animal sector in the region is currently not as well provided with diagnostic and professional health services as the livestock sector. Member Countries see an increasing role for health professionals (veterinarians and others) in their country,

In some Member Countries, fisheries authorities have either the sole responsibility for aquatic animal health or share it with the Veterinary Services. In these countries, fisheries authorities would take the lead in mounting an emergency response to an aquatic animal disease outbreak, and the Veterinary Services are usually well experienced in managing terrestrial animal emergency disease outbreaks, but there is infrequent contact between the two,

In many Member Countries, draft texts for the Aquatic Code and the Aquatic Manual reach aquatic animal health experts either too late or not at all, resulting in few official comments. This means that Member Countries do not sufficiently use the opportunity to influence the setting of international standards that underpin international trade,

Fundamental changes to the Aquatic Code and Aquatic Manual have been adopted in 2003. These include the listing of aquatic animal diseases and the requirements for reporting on the status of listed diseases. It is important that Member Countries fully understand these new arrangements and accept and fulfil their obligations on disease reporting,

Most Member Countries provide annual and quarterly aquatic animal disease reports, but there are numerous reporting errors such as the use of inappropriate symbols; the provision of conflicting information to the OIE's Tokyo Office and to the Central Bureau; and not reporting new disease occurrences that would be of major epidemiological significance to other countries in the region,

The OIE continues to engage in regional aquatic animal health initiatives, together with the FAO and NACA, but enhanced involvement of both veterinary and fisheries authorities within Member Countries is required to achieve the desired outcomes in areas such as improving Member Countries' knowledge of OIE standard-setting activities in the field of aquatic animal health and the transparency of epidemiological reporting.

THE REGIONAL COMMISSION FOR ASIA, THE FAR EAST AND OCEANIA RECOMMENDS:

A) THAT THE OIE:

1. Reinforce to Delegates their responsibility to the OIE for terrestrial as well as aquatic animals.
2. Encourage Member Countries to strengthen veterinary and other tertiary education in aquatic animal health.
3. Request Member Countries to clarify the roles and responsibilities for aquatic animal health assigned to veterinary and other authorities in their country.
4. Provide opportunities to assist cooperation between veterinary and other authorities responsible for aquatic animal health in Member Countries, for example, by inviting other authorities to attend OIE-sponsored conferences/workshops that have an aquatic theme.
5. Direct efforts at increasing general awareness with national Delegates world-wide about, for example, the provisions of the Aquatic Code and Aquatic Manual.
6. Request the Aquatic Animal Commission to provide regular updates of the Aquatic Code and Aquatic Manual at Regional Commission Conferences or other suitable venues.
7. Direct efforts at obtaining more comments on draft texts for the Aquatic Code and Aquatic Manual from a larger number of national Delegates, for example, consider from the Delegates of Member Countries the nomination of an 'aquatic national focal point' as a parallel recipient of Aquatic Animal Commission reports on behalf of national Delegates.

8. Provide Member Countries with the necessary assistance and guidance on accurate, timely and effective aquatic animal disease reporting.
9. Continue to cooperate with relevant international and regional organisations to increase awareness about aquatic animal health in the region, to improve disease reporting and to foster cooperation between veterinary and fisheries authorities within countries.

B) THAT THE MEMBER COUNTRIES:

1. Direct efforts at improving the coverage of the aquatic sectors with health services and strengthen veterinary and other tertiary education in aquatic animal health.
2. Clarify the roles and responsibilities for aquatic animal health assigned to veterinary and other authorities in their country.
3. Request their Veterinary Services to improve the communication and cooperation with fishery authorities, especially regarding disease reporting and disease emergency responses.
4. Where primary responsibility for aquatic animal health rests with an authority other than the Veterinary Services, nominate an 'aquatic national focal point' from the other authority, so that the OIE may circulate Aquatic Animal Commission reports to the 'aquatic national focal point' at the same time as when circulating to national Delegates (providing comments back to the OIE must take place through, and with the endorsement of, the national Delegate to the OIE).
5. Significantly enhance circulation of draft texts for the Aquatic Code and Aquatic Manual amongst experts, and provide comments through the national Delegate to the OIE.
6. Significantly improve the quality of aquatic animal disease reports, and request the OIE's assistance where clarification is needed.

(Adopted by the OIE Regional Commission for Asia, the Far East and Oceania on 28 November 2003 and endorsed by the International Committee of the OIE on 27 May 2004)

Fig. 1: The "Nouméa Recommendations", adopted by the OIE Regional Commission for Asia, the Far East and Oceania on 28 November 2003 and endorsed by the International Committee of the OIE on 27 May 2004

Among the "Nouméa Recommendations" are that the OIE *"reinforce to Delegates their responsibility to the OIE for terrestrial as well as aquatic animals"; "request Member Countries to clarify the roles and responsibilities for aquatic animal health assigned to veterinary and other authorities in their country"; and "provide opportunities to assist cooperation between veterinary and other authorities responsible for aquatic animal health in Member Countries…".*

Concluding Remarks

This OIE Conference provides an opportunity to assist the OIE and its Member Countries in exchanging the latest information on developing a science-based approach to the management of aquatic animal health and welfare, and to present the valuable experience gained in the past few years. The presentations have been selected to assist in the evaluation and improvement of the current standards and guidelines for better control of aquatic animal infections and of countries' capabilities to prepare for, and respond to, aquatic animal disease emergencies. They will also assist in better defining roles and responsibilities.

References

1 FAO: State of world aquaculture 2006. FAO Fisheries Technical Paper. No 500. Rome, FAO. 2006. 134pp. (Accessed 22 December 2006 from http://www.fao.org/newsroom/en/news/2006/1000383/index.html).

2 Bernoth EM: Update on developments in aquatic animal diseases, in OIE: Compendium on Technical Items presented to the International Committee or Regional Commissions. OIE, Paris, 2004, pp 161-183.

3 23rd Conference of the OIE Regional Commission for Asia, the Far East and Oceania, Nouméa (New Caledonia), 25-28 November 2003: Recommendation No. 2: Update on developments in aquatic animal diseases, in OIE: Final Report 2004. 72nd General Session, Paris, 23-28 May 2004. OIE, Paris, 2004, pp 169-171. (Accessed 22 December 2006 from http://www.oie.int/eng/OIE/actes/en_rfinal.htm).

Dr. Eva-Maria Bernoth, DMV, President, OIE Aquatic Animal Health StandardsCommission, c/o Office of the Chief Veterinary Officer, Australian Government Department of Agriculture, Fisheries and Forestry, GPO Box 858, Canberra ACT 2601, Australia.
E-mail: Eva-Maria.Bernoth@daff.gov.au

Dodet B, the OIE Scientific & Technical Department (eds): The OIE Global Conference on Aquatic Animal Healths. Dev Biol (Basel). Basel, Karger, 2007, vol 129, p 11.

Session II

Cooperation among Stakeholders in Aquatic Animal Disease Management

Chairperson: *E.-M. Bernoth*, Australia

Dodet B, the OIE Scientific & Technical Department (eds):The OIE Global Conference on Aquatic Animal Health. Dev Biol (Basel). Basel, Karger, 2007, vol 129, pp 13-19.

Cooperation between Veterinary and Fisheries Authorities in Aquatic Animal Management in Sri Lanka

S.K.R. Amarasekara

Director General, Department of Animal Production and Health, Gatambe, Peradeniya Sri Lanka

Key words: aquatic animal management, Sri Lanka, Veterinary Authorities, cooperation

Abstract: The need for effective cooperation between the Veterinary and Fisheries Authorities in the field of aquatic animal health is widely accepted in Sri Lanka. International organisations have requested Sri Lanka to develop a model to promote this cooperation. With no tradition of aquaculture, Sri Lanka ventured into commercial aquaculture only a few decades ago. Epizootic ulcerative syndrome (EUS), monodon baculovirus and white spot syndrome virus are the only OIE recognized diseases reported.

Responsibility for disease diagnosis, the implementation of preventive and control measures and certification is held by three institutions: the National Aquaculture Development Authority (NAQDA), the National Aquatic Research and Development Agency (NARA) and the Department of Animal Production and Health (DAPH). The National Centre for Disease Diagnosis and Health Management in Aquaculture is at the University of Peradeniya. The Fisheries and Aquatic Resources Act (No.2 of 1996), the Animal Diseases Act (No. 59 of 1992), the Animal Feeds Act of 1986 and the Aquaculture Management (Disease Control) Regulations 2000 provide the legislative framework for aquatic health issues. Coordination among the institutions involved in aquatic health management is inadequate and there is no proper policy and strategy for promoting aquatic health. Surveillance programs and epidemiological studies are also inadequate.

A new structure has been proposed for better coordination between Veterinary and Fisheries Authorities in Sri Lanka to encourage all stakeholders in aquatic health control to participate in a coordinated effort. This new initiative will not only promote cooperation between Veterinary and Fisheries authorities but also strengthen the national aquatic animal health network.

Introduction

Veterinary and Fisheries cooperation in the field of aquatic animal health is an important subject which is currently widely discussed. It has been discussed at OIE meetings as well as the FAO consultations and at the 3rd and 4th Asia Regional Advisory Group meetings held in Thailand and Sri Lanka. The international organisations have requested Sri Lanka to develop a model in this field especially because of the high level of cooperation between Sri Lankan Veterinary and Fisheries Authorities.

The Development of Aquaculture and Fish Disease Management

Sri Lanka is a small country with a total land area of 65,000 km2 and a coastal belt around 1,500 km long. Historically, Sri Lanka has no traditional aquaculture even though there is traditional fishing in coastal areas. Since 1951, the government has tried to develop the aquaculture industry through the introduction of exotic fish species. Culture based fisheries in seasonal tanks were introduced in the mid- and late eighties, and have become a major component of aquaculture today under the Aquaculture Resources Development and Quality Improvement Project (ARDQUIP) funded by the Asian Development Bank (ADB) and implemented by the Ministry of Fisheries, Aquatic Resources and Christian Affairs (MFARCA).

Ornamental fish culture on a commercial scale began in the mid-seventies, when Sri Lanka opted for an open economy, while the development of the shrimp industry on a commercial scale began in the mid-eighties. Unpolluted water bodies, a high level of biodiversity, and increasing local and export market demand encouraged the expansion of aquaculture. Sri Lanka earned a good reputation for quality farmed and wild caught fish in international markets and aquaculture thus became a valuable export industry, providing many employment opportunities. Earnings from the export of ornamental fish reached Rs. 623 million in 2003, an increase of 18% over 2002 [1]. Aquarium fish exports from Sri Lanka are increasing annually at a growth rate of 16.9 % [2]. The USA was the biggest importer in 2002, followed by Japan, the United Kingdom and Germany, respectively. Sri Lanka fulfills approximately 1% of the total world demand for ornamental fish [3]. Shrimp exportation was at 1,800 metric tons in 2005, earning 1,769 million rupees. The major markets were Japan and the USA.

Sri Lanka's ornamental fish industry consists of a wide variety of fish species from fresh water, marine and brackish water environments. The marine sector comprises captive fish species from the sea. Of the fresh water species, the guppy (*Poecilia reticulata*) ranks the highest with 67% of total exports, followed by swordtails (family *Xiphiidae*), angels (*Pterophyllum scalare*) and platys (Xiphophorus *sp.*)[4]. *Penaeus monodon* is the major shrimp species cultured in Sri Lanka. Before culture technology was introduced, total production came from wild capture. Substantial amounts of production and broodstock for hatcheries is still supplied by the captive fisheries.

The aquaculture industry is a fast moving import and export trade. Outbreaks of different diseases have not been rare in the recent past. Diseases are one of the major factors that determine the world market demand, and their prevention, diagnosis, control and treatment have therefore become very important issues.

Diseases affecting shrimp and ornamental fish may have a bacterial, viral, fungal or parasitic origin. These diseases are a real threat to a sustainable industry. Bacterial diseases are caused mainly by Gram-negative bacteria including *Aeromonas hydropila* [5], *Vibrio sp.* [6] and *Flexibacter columnaris* [7].

Epizootic ulcerative syndrome (EUS) is a seasonal fungal disease condition that usually occurs after heavy rains and during the cooler period of the year. The causative agent is *Aphanomyces invaderis* [5]. This disease was reported in Sri Lanka in the late eighties as a massive outbreak. Until EUS was reported, OIE listed diseases had not been recorded in ornamental or food fish in Sri Lanka. Now the incidence is rare. In addition to *Aphanomyces invaderis, Saprolegnia sp. and Achlya sp.* are present in the country.

Parasitic diseases are the main fish diseases in Sri Lanka, and include *Ichtyobodo, Cryptobia, Hexamita, Piscinoodinium/Amylodinium, Ichthyophthirius multifilis, Trichodina sp., Chilodonella, Tetrahymena. Capillaria sp., Gyrodactylus sp., Dactylogyrus sp., Centrocestus sp., Argulus sp., Learnea sp.* and *Ergasilus sp.*. The *Tetrahymena* from the epidemic in 1998 was named the guppy killer disease [8]. Recently there have been no parasitic disease outbreaks.

There are records of two major viral diseases in the country, namely those caused by Monodon baculovirus (MBV) and White spot syndrome virus (WSSV). MBV first appeared in 1988 and now it is endemic in wild stocks. Disease incidence is low at present. WSSV was first reported in 1996 [9]. Both are OIE listed diseases but WSSV disease has posed the greatest threat to the shrimp industry of Sri Lanka.

Organizations Involved in Aquatic Animal Health Management

Disease diagnosis in aquatic organisms and the implementation of preventive measures is the responsibility of the National Aquatic Development Authority (NAQDA) and the National Aquatic Resources and Development Agency (NARA), both under the purview of the MFARCA. Certification of live fish exports and imports to and from all countries for the ornamental fish industry, to countries other than the European Union for the processed sea food industry, is however, the responsibility of the Department of Animal production and Health (DAPH) under the purview of the Ministry of Estate Infrastructure and Livestock (MEIL) of Sri Lanka. Occurrences of viral, bacterial, fungal and parasitic diseases in the aquaculture sector (shrimp, edible fish and ornamental fish) have been reported from time to time by researchers at universities and research institutions. Presently, there are shrimp farm extension and monitoring officers and regional aquaculture extension officers (similar to inspectors) attached to the NAQDA who have been trained to report disease incidences in aquaculture. Veterinary Investigation Centres (VIC) are also being established in each district of the country to investigate into the field situation, while the national universities conduct graduate and postgraduate degree programmes with modules in aquatic animal health management and disease diagnosis for both Veterinary and Fisheries Officers.

Aquatic animal health issues have mainly been in the hands of departments and agencies under the purview of the MFARCA for about three decades. However, the country has now recognized that Veterinary Authorities in the DAPH should play a lead role in meeting OIE requirements, while maintaining cordial relationships and good cooperation with Fisheries Authorities when dealing with aquatic animal health management activities. As most of the veterinarians in Sri Lanka have limited training in aquatic animal health, initially they may have to depend to some extent on trained personnel attached to other institutions in the country. It may also be pertinent to mention that during recent years several BVSc graduates, well trained in aquatic animal health, have been recruited by the DAPH.

Meanwhile, the ARDQUIP of the MFARCA has identified the need for a national centre for disease diagnosis and health management in aquaculture. Thus the Centre for Aquatic Animal Disease Diagnosis and Research (CAADDR) is being established at the Faculty of Veterinary Medicine and Animal Science, at the University of Peradeniya. It is envisaged that this centre will play a vital role in facilitating the tasks of NAQDA, which is empowered with the responsibility of developing sustainable aquaculture in Sri Lanka while promoting more active cooperation among Veterinary and Aquaculture/Fisheries Authorities.

LEGAL PROVISIONS

In Sri Lanka adequate legal provisions exist to effectively cover aquatic health management. The two most important acts are the Fisheries and Aquatic Resources Act (No.2 of 1996) administered by the Department of Fisheries and Aquatic Resources (DFAR), and the Animal Diseases Act (No.59 of 1992) administered by the DAPH. There is other legislation such as the Animal Feeds Act of 1986 and the regulations published under the Fisheries and Aquatic Resources Act cited as the Aquaculture Management (Disease Control) Regulations 2000, which facilitates interventions in aquatic health issues.

The most important provisions in the Fisheries and Aquatic Resources Act are stipulations that no aquaculture farm can be set up without a license from DFAR and that DFAR has the authority to close farms in the event of a disease outbreak. The Animal Diseases Act and the regulations framed under it provide for the DAPH to take appropriate measures to control animal diseases. The definition of animal includes aquatic animals. The DAPH also makes provisions to prevent the entry of animal diseases into Sri Lanka through the animal quarantine system. Another important legal provision in this Act is the authority to control the use of drugs and biological products against animal diseases.

The DAPH has several divisions, each headed by a Director. The three divisions involved in fisheries activities are the Animal Health Division, the Veterinary Research Division and the Regulatory Division. The animal quarantine system under the Regulatory Division comprises the animal quarantine service at the main sea port as well as the airport, providing a 24 hour service. Export and import certification is their responsibility. The VIC at district level operates under the Animal Health Division. The VIC at Welisara carries out bacterial and parasitic disease diagnosis as well as water quality testing. The specialised laboratories situated at the Veterinary Research Institute have the capability to carry out the diagnosis of viral and other specific diseases.

Certification Process for Aquatic Items

For over a decade the DAPH has been involved in the export certification of ornamental fish (annual export is around US$7 M). The EU and Japan require the export certification of the DFAR for shrimp, live lobsters, live crabs, fresh chilled fish, frozen fish, crab meat, and lobster. Export certification of these products for other countries is done by the DAPH. The pre-export quarantine inspection and testing requirement varies from country to country. Depending on the country, the quarantine period varies from seven to 30 days. Most countries require an aquatic health certification covering all OIE listed diseases.

Import Procedure

Imports of aquaculture products and frozen fish products into Sri Lanka require an import approval from the DAPH. The import approvals depend entirely on the international veterinary certificate issued by the exporting country to cover all OIE listed aquatic animal diseases. The import procedures for aquaculture products are available at the Animal Quarantine Station, and all importers have been made aware of them. All imported aquaculture items must undergo inspection and testing during the surveillance period before release. DAPH is in the process of developing an aquatic animal disease protocol which would require a specified international veterinary certificate to accompany imported aquatic items.

Constraints in Aquatic Health Management

There are several major constraints in the aquatic animal health management system. DAPH is under the purview of the MEIL while DFAR and other institutions of the fisheries sector come under the purview of the MFARCR. Since two different Ministries are involved, policy decisions are either delayed or inconsistent. In addition, there is no proper policy and strategy for aquatic health management in Sri Lanka. Furthermore, coordination among the institutions involved in aquatic health management is inadequate. Thus, the institutions operate in isolation without focusing on a common goal, unlike with terrestrial animal health management, where responsibility lies with the DAPH. These shortcomings are due to inadequate infrastructure facilities. To ensure a satisfactory level of aquatic animal health, the scattered resources need to be pooled and used efficiently with a definite role for each organisation, including the private sector.

Another constraint is the lack of trained manpower. Adequately trained manpower is urgently required. More and more local training as well as sufficient foreign training is required to achieve the targets. Assistance should be sought from funding organizations in this area.

A further limitation is the inadequacy of positions in government institutions. One suggestion to ease the situation is to encourage and involve the private sector in specific areas of aquatic health management such as laboratory services, data collection and the dissemination of information.

Disease Reporting

Aquatic disease information is collected regularly on the basis of the NACA and OIE lists of diseases. The passive and active surveillance programmes for aquatic animal diseases in Sri Lanka are at the basic level. Similarly, only a few epidemiological studies have been carried out in this field. Therefore these areas need to be strengthened, along with other aspects of disease reporting.

Sri Lanka has appointed a National Coordinator from NAQDA while the National Focal Point is appointed from the NARA. They gather disease information from Research Centres as well as Aquatic Resource Centres in the prescribed format. The information is forwarded to the NACA as well as to the OIE through Director General of the DAPH, since he is the country delegate to the OIE.

The Proposed Aquatic Animal Health Disease Reporting Structure

A new structure has been proposed to achieve effective aquatic animal disease reporting and for better coordination between Veterinary and Fisheries Authorities in Sri Lanka. The salient feature of this proposal is to encourage all stakeholders in aquatic animal disease control to participate in a coordinated effort with a specific role for each organization. This effort has yet to be tested. Embarking on this kind of new initiative will not only promote cooperation between Veterinary and Fisheries Authorities, but will also strengthen the national aquatic animal health network. Furthermore this will make effective use of the existing information and improve communication between stakeholders.

The Proposed National Advisory Committee on Aquatic Animal Health

A national body on aquatic animal health is currently needed to address all major issues in this field. Therefore it has been proposed that a National Advisory Committee on Aquatic Animal Health be established. The main function will be to advise the Government on national issues, policy and strategies. The proposed committee may comprise representatives from the two Ministries (Fisheries and Livestock), regulatory bodies, research organizations, and industry and trade partners. This body could also coordinate the activities of the institutions involved in aquatic animal health.

References

1 Central Bank of Sri Lanka. Annual Report 2003.

2 Ekarathne SUK: A Review of the status and treads of exported ornamental fish resources and their habitat in Sri Lanka. Bay of Bengal Program BOPH/REP/88, Chennai, 2003, pp 3-8.

3 Haputhnathri H, Perera PAJC, Vidanage SP: Development of ornamental fish production and culture for increased export earnings and employment opportunities in Sri Lanka. Socio economic and market research division, National Aquatic Research Development Agency, Sri Lanka, 1998, pp 4-11.

4 Haputhnathri H,

5 Chandrakanthi WHS, Pathiratne A, Widanapathirana S: Characteristics and virulence of Aeromonas hydrophila isolates from freshwater fish with epizootic ulcerative syndrome (EUS). J Natl Science Found Sri Lanka 2000;28 (1): 29-42.

6 Vasantha GKH, Hettiarachchi M: Pathogencity of fresh water Vibrio sp. on ornamental fish Pterophyllum scalare. Proceedings of the 51st Annual Section Association for the Adv Science Sri Lanka, 1995, pp 272-274.

7 Hettiarachchi M, Hettiarachchi DC: A study on columnaris disease in the guppy, Poecilia reticulate. Proceedings of the 5th symposium on Disease in Asian Aquaculture Queensland, Australia, 1995, p.116.

8 Thilakaratne IDSIP, Rajapakse G, Hewakopura A, Rajapakse RPVJ, Fizal ACM.

9 Some parasites associated with ornamental fish in Sri Lanka; a preliminary Investigation. Proceedings of the 52nd Annual Convention of Sri Lanka Veterinary Association; Sri Lanka Vet J, 2000;47-62.

10 Siriwardena PPGSN: Management strategies for major diseases in shrimp aquaculture in Sri Lanka. Country paper presented at the FAO/NACA/WWF International Workshop on Management Strategies for Major Diseases in Shrimp Aquaculture, Thailand 1999.

Dr. Sri Kamal Ranjith Amarasekara, Director General, Department of Animal Production and Health, Getambe, Peradeniya, Sri Lanka
E-mail: dgaphamara@sltnet.lk

Dodet B, the OIE Scientific & Technical Department (eds): The OIE Global Conference on Aquatic Animal Health. Dev Biol (Basel). Basel, Karger, 2007, vol 129, pp 21-28.

Managing the Koi Herpesvirus Disease Outbreak in Indonesia and the Lessons Learned

M.G. Bondad-Reantaso[1], A. Sunarto[2], R.P. Subasinghe[1]

1 Department of Fisheries and Aquaculture, Food and Agriculture Organization of the United Nations (FAO), Viale delle Terme di Caracalla, 00100 Rome, Italy

2 Fish Health Research Laboratory, Jl. Ragunan 20, Pasar Minggu, Jakarta 12540, Indonesia

Key words: akoi herpesvirus (KHV), Indonesia, outbreak, epizootic

Abstract: In 2002, the suspected koi herpesvirus (KHV) outbreak in Indonesia was investigated by an International Emergency Disease Control Task Force organized by NACA immediately following a request for assistance by the Government of Indonesia. The Task Force gained immediate support from ACIAR, AAHRI, FAO, CENTEX-Thailand, INTERVET, Stirling University, and the University of California. The Task Force findings revealed the involvement of an infectious agent, an analogy with KHV outbreaks, its introduction through fish importation and its spread into other areas through fish movement.

A number of actions taken by the Government of Indonesia included temporary restrictions, through a Ministry Circular, on the movement of koi and common carps, intensive information dissemination, emergency notification to the OIE, and early warning to neighbouring countries. FAO immediately responded by providing an emergency technical assistance project to improve Indonesia's national capacity to respond to the carp disease epizootic.

Recognizing the significance of and necessity for: (a) enhancing regional and international cooperation;(b) improving awareness of emerging disease epizootics and improving diagnostic capabilities at both national and regional levels;(c) proactive reporting of serious disease outbreaks as a mechanism for early warning;(d) detailed documentation of outbreak scenarios;(e) emergency preparedness;(f) empowering farmers to manage disease and other risks; and (g) strong national commitment from concerned authorities are some of the important lessons learned. Despite the intense efforts, the spread of KHV did not stop and continued to affect other countries such as Japan, China, the Taiwan Province of the Republic of China, and most recently Thailand. All relevant stakeholders cannot afford to be complacent and we need innovative responses to current and future disease challenges. The lessons learned in managing the Indonesian KHV outbreak as well as lessons from past disease epizootics will hopefully assist us in improving preparedness and responses to similar events when they occur in the future.

Introduction

During the 12th Governing Council Meeting of the Network of Aquaculture Centres in Asia-Pacific (NACA) held in Malaysia in January, 2002, a Hungarian colleague inquired whether there was a certain carp disease affecting Asia. This prompted the collection of relevant information which lead to come across a disease known as koi herpesvirus (KHV). In April 2002, during the World Aquaculture Society meeting (WAS 2002) in Beijing, China, an Israeli plenary speaker talked about KHV and predicted that it would only be a matter of time before KHV hits Asia. It was not yet known at that time that there was already an ongoing disease outbreak in Indonesia. In June, 2002, an urgent phone call from Indonesia sought assistance from NACA concerning a serious disease of cyprinids. NACA suspected it to be KHV based on the description of the clinical signs and patterns of mortality. During the National Strategy Workshop, organized by NACA, Israeli material presented by the author and the Indonesian presentation based on the ongoing outbreak were indistinguishable; the earlier suspicion of KHV proved correct [1].

In June-July, 2002, the suspected koi herpesvirus (KHV) outbreak in Indonesia was investigated by an International Emergency Disease Control Task Force organized by NACA immediately following a request for technical assistance by the Government of Indonesia. The Task Force gained immediate support from the Australian Centre for International Agricultural Research (ACIAR), the Aquatic Animal Health Research Institute (AAHRI) of Thailand's Department of Fisheries, the Food and Agriculture Organization of the United Nations (FAO), CENTEX-Thailand, INTERVET, the Stirling University, and the University of California.

This paper presents some of the important achievements and lessons learned in managing the KHV outbreak in Indonesia.

Major Findings and Achievements of the International Emergency Disease Control Task Force

In March, 2002, a serious disease outbreak affecting koi and common carp populations occurred in Indonesia, in the area of Blitar in East Java. An International Emergency Disease Control Task Force organized by NACA composed of an epidemiologist, a virologist and an aquatic animal health specialist travelled to Indonesia to investigate the disease situation, establish a case definition of the disease in question, collect relevant information, collect samples for laboratory analysis, and generate specific recommendations for the Government of Indonesia and regional measures to prevent the further spread of the disease. The general direction of the Task Force investigation was to determine the possible involvement of KHV based on preliminary observations available at that time [2].

The Task Force findings revealed a very close analogy with KHV outbreaks elsewhere. These include observations such as sudden onset, rapid spread, specificity to koi and common carp, and spread into other areas through fish movements. The clinical signs, consistent in all cases, included bronchial hemorrhage, necrosis and focal dermal ulceration. The level of morbidity and mortality reported by farmers ranged from 50 to 100%. Water temperatures, suggested to be a principal environmental factor influencing the severity and onset of KHV infection, ranged from 19-23°C during the outbreak period [1].

The work of the Task Force revealed that although an infectious agent was involved, the aetiological agent (suspected to be KHV) could not be confirmed due to the absence of typical KHV pathology, failed viral isolation and non-observance of the typical virions through electron microscopy. Nevertheless, the Task Force work provided supportive evidence of possible KHV association as KHV was detected by polymerase chain reaction (PCR) from all case samples, indicating that KHV may have played a role in the observed mortalities. Since the outbreak in question was a first time diagnosis of a very serious disease, it was considered essential that all available diagnostic techniques (e.g. pathology, viral isolation, PCR, in-situ hybridization and electron microscopy) be used by the Task Force to confirm the causative agent. Because KHV involvement could not be confirmed, it was thought best to call this serious outbreak "Mass Mortality of Koi and Common Carp" at that point in time.

The most important achievements of the Task Force included a quick response to the request for technical assistance through convening of the International Emergency Disease Control Task Force; provision of supporting evidence on the association of KHV with the outbreak in question [2,3]; recommendation for immediate notification of the outbreak to the OIE, reported as suspected KHV and later named as Mass Mortality of Koi and Common Carp [4]; providing early warning to neighbouring countries and intensive information dissemination; and provision of relevant information which formed the basis for the development of a 3-year emergency technical assistance project through FAO's Technical Cooperation Programme [2].

Subsequent Findings under the FAO Technical Cooperation Project TCP/INS/2905 "Health Management in Freshwater Aquaculture in Indonesia"

The Task Force did not confirm the exact aetiology of the observed mortalities however the initial observations, findings and recommendations became the basis for the development of the FAO Technical Cooperation Project TCP/INS/2905 "Health management in freshwater aquaculture in Indonesia." Subsequent work under this FAO project confirmed that the 2002 outbreak was indeed caused by KHV, based on a more detailed epidemiological survey and diagnostic assessment of subsequent disease outbreaks [5].

The 3-year FAO TCP project was aimed at addressing the following concerns: institutional strengthening and capacity building; a national strategy on aquatic animal health; legislation; surveillance and reporting; viral disease diagnostic laboratories; a national epidemiological survey of KHV; information systems; and training of government staff and farmers.

The FAO TCP made many important achievements. It confirmed KHV as the causative agent of subsequent outbreaks, based on a more detailed epidemiological survey and diagnostic assessment of subsequent disease outbreaks. It also determined the extent of spread of the disease with documented episodes of 10 major KHV outbreaks in Indonesia, identified risk areas and conducted a retrospective analysis of the origin of KHV in Indonesia. The first episode originated from the first outbreak in Blitar in East Java from infected koi carp. It then spread to aquacultured common carp and eventually other natural bodies such as lakes and rivers in Java and Sumatra. Based on quarantine records in Surabaya, it was revealed that koi carps were imported from China through Hong Kong. This batch of koi carp were transferred from Surabaya to Blitar. Blitar is the centre of production for koi in Indonesia. Some of these Blitar koi were transferred to Bandung in East Java which then had an outbreak immediately after. Neighbouring Subang - a major centre for common carp production - had an outbreak in March-April, 2002. As infected fish were being moved from Subang, KHV spread to the Cirata reservoir affecting both cultured and wild carps. Even as a Ministerial Decree was issued in June, 2002, restricting live fish movement, KHV continued to spread now affecting the island of Sumatra. By end of 2005, there were unconfirmed reports of KHV occurrence in Sentani Lake in the West Papua Province. It was confirmed that the outbreak in West Papua was KHV.

The FAO TCP developed containment and contingency plans which were implemented and led to a reduction in further losses. These included strong enforcement of the ban on inter-island movement of koi carp supported by enhanced cooperation with breeders, traders and the general public; prevention of further movement of the disease northwards into Sumatra and any spread into Sulawesi and Kalimantan; establishment of disease free zones, particularly on the island of Java, through effective farm level biosecurity; continuous reporting and surveillance of disease as a basis for implementing the ban; and an enhanced awareness program on general health management, diseases risks and promotion of good health management practices.

The project improved the disease diagnostic capacity of the state laboratories. A National Virology Unit was established at the Fish Health Research Laboratory (FHRL), including provision of basic equipment and training of staff, with capacity to do fish viral isolation, transport samples, maintain cell lines, culture viruses from fish, grow and maintain a small virus reference collection and produce primary fish cell cultures. Towards the end of project implementation, the Indonesians were successful in isolating the KHV virus.

Human resources were developed through various training activities provided to fish health personnel from the state agency. Numerous training workshops were undertaken under the TCP on various aspects of aquatic animal health management (including laboratory based training) conducted by national and international consultants. Attendance at overseas technical training programmes at AAHRI and a number of overseas seminars/conferences/meetings was made possible and greatly upgraded the technical skills of some of the project staff members.

The FAO TCP also paved the way for the organization of a Regional Workshop on Preparedness and Response to Aquatic Animal Health Emergencies in Asia which reviewed regional experiences in responding to disease emergencies including the work in the FAO TCP [6] and the publication of guidelines for preparedness and response to aquatic animal health emergencies in Asia [7].

Lesson Learned from Managing the KHV Outbreak in Indonesia

KHV is a classical example of a disease that originated in an ornamental fish and spread to cultured fish and wild fisheries. The KHV outbreak in Indonesia is yet another strong piece evidence of ornamental fish as a significant vector for viral diseases (along with Spring viremia of carp and ranaviruses). The ornamental fish trade is unregulated. Within the context of trade – this calls for a change in the current thinking - how to deal with ornamentals. Responsible trading of live aquatics through effective or meaningful import health requirements is essential.

The various lessons learned from managing the KHV outbreak in Indonesia are elaborated below.

The importance of regional and international cooperation

The Emergency Task Force was a rapid coordinated effort and a critical quick action that triggered a chain of events for an immediate investigation of the outbreak and garnered tremendous support from development aid/scientific groups. These events included preliminary diagnosis, establishment of a case definition, implementation of specific actions and control measures at a national level, and early warning for neighbouring countries and trading partners of Indonesia. The initial findings became the basis for emergency technical assistance from FAO.

Other actions taken at the regional/international level included convening three major conferences on KHV: the International Workshop on KHV, London, UK, February, 2004 (OATA/CEFAS); the International Conference on KHV, Yokohama, Japan, March, 2004 (Fisheries Agency of Japan); and the Expert Workshop on Emergency Preparedness and Response to Aquatic Animal Diseases in Asia, Indonesia, September, 2004 (FAO). KHV became such a high profile disease that it called for three major conferences on the same subject within a year – this was unprecedented.

Enhancing awareness of emerging epizootics and improving diagnostic capacities at both national and regional levels

The Asian region has experienced many disease emergencies over the last three decades. All relevant stakeholders cannot afford to be complacent and there is a need for innovative responses to current and future disease challenges. It is important to enhance awareness of emerging disease epizootics in other regions. Improving diagnostics is also a key element and there will be more need for epidemiologists, pathologists and risk analysts.

Proactive reporting of serious disease outbreaks as a mechanism for early warning

The first meeting of the NACA's Regional Advisory Group, in November, 2002, recommended the inclusion of 'Koi Mass Mortality' under the category of 'Unknown diseases of serious nature' and the Second Meeting strongly recommended to direct efforts at improving surveillance and reporting of this disease. Subsequently, Hong Kong SAR, Japan, Thailand, Singapore and Philippines immediately initiated a surveillance programme for KHV.

The importance of detailed documentation

In the case of the Indonesian outbreak, the detailed documentation (Task Force report, OIE notification, technical reports, mission reports, scientific publications, memorandum circulars, etc.) became permanent records of the series of events, findings and actions taken and served as a valuable reference point for making a retrospective analysis of the origin of KHV in Indonesia, providing early warning information to neighbouring and trading partners of Indonesia. Examples of the documents produced were the NACA/ACIAR Report [2], the epidemiology section of the Task Force Report by Cameron [3], the OIE Notification by Rukyani [4], Trans-boundary Aquatic Animal Diseases: focus on Koi herpesvirus (KHV) by Bondad-Reantaso [1], Review of KHV by Bondad-Reantaso and Subasinghe [8], the paper on field investigations on KHV by Sunarto et al [5], the paper on viral isolation by Sunarto et al [9] and a few others [10-12].

Emergency preparedness

In terms of economic losses and investment, Table 1 below shows an increasing trend in the losses from the first outbreak in Blitar up to the most recent major outbreak ranging from US$ 0.5 to US$ 25 M. This table also shows an overview of examples of investment provided to assist in better understanding and managing the disease.

Examples of losses	Examples of investment
The Blitar March, 2002, outbreak: US$ 0.5 M Up to the July, 2002, outbreak: US$ 5 M	NACA Emergency Disease Task Force: US$ 20,000 FAO TCP: US$ 325,000
Up to the December, 2002/2003, outbreak: US$ 10 M /US$ 15 M	Government of Indonesia internal budget: US$ 200,000
Up to the November, 2004, outbreak: US$ 25 M	Japanese Trust Fund: US$ 20,000 (for research)

From this single case alone, we can see that there is a huge amount of money involved both in terms of losses and investments. The losses incurred could have been more had it not been for a speedy response. The NACA Task Force was an ad hoc action but nevertheless could very well serve as a model. There needs to be, however, some institutionalized mechanism in terms of an expert group, funding and other required resources to deal with aquatic animal disease emergencies. It is particularly important to know how to deal with 'unknown diseases'. Having a reference laboratory for exotic diseases at both national and regional levels will be essential. Dealing with an emergency disease situation therefore calls for effective regional and international cooperation and putting emergency preparedness with advanced planning as a core function of an appropriately mandated institution.

Empowering farmers to manage disease and other risks

In order to deal with day-to-day situations in farms, pond/farm health management is crucial to preventing, controlling and even eradicating serious disease. Inequities in aquatic animal medicine and/or husbandry education as well as inaccurate information dissemination are core issues. Empowering with information and tools such as better aquaculture management practices (e.g., good farm hygiene such as hand washing between tanks, separation of nets/tanks/stocks, maintaining good water quality, proper handling of fish and good record keeping, for example, gross and environmental observations and stoking records including movement records of fish in and out of the facility) or simple and practical biosecurity measures at the farm level (e.g., proper quarantine of incoming fish, removal of dead fish from ponds, drying and liming of ponds, regular and correct disinfection procedures, and the exclusion of wild fish) are all essential in understanding the disease situation at the farm level. Educating farmers and hobbyists on good health management and responsible trading of live aquatic animals is the key to disease prevention and early warning/reporting is the key to minimize disease spread [8].

Strong National Commitment from Concerned Authorities

Another important lesson is having a strong commitment from national authorities. In the case of Indonesia, this was manifested through the continued support to KHV investigation even after completion of the external assistance through such activities as surveillance and reporting, continuation of the aquatic animal information system and full support to the virology laboratory.

References

1 Bondad-Reantaso MG: Trans-boundary aquatic animal diseases: focus on Koi herpesvirus (KHV). Aquaculture Asia 2004;IX(2):24-28.

2 NACA/ACIAR: Report of emergency disease control task force on a serious disease of koi and common carps in Indonesia. NACA, Bangkok, 2002.

3 Cameron A: Report of an epidemiological investigation of a serious outbreak of disease amongst koi and common carp in Indonesia. Report prepared for the Emergency Disease Control Task Force on a Serious Disease of Koi and Common Carps in Indonesia. NACA, Bangkok, 2002.

4 Rukyani A: Koi herpesvirus in Indonesia: suspicion. Report of KHV epidemic to OIE, 2002 (available at www.oie.int).

5 Sunarto A, Taukhid, Rukyani A, Koesharyani I, Supriyadi H, Gardenia L, Huminto H, Agungpriyono DR, Pasaribu FH, Widodo, Herdikiawan D, Rukmono D, Prayitno SB: Field investigations on a serious disease outbreak among koi and common carp (Cyprinus carpio) in Indonesial, in Walker PJ, Lester RG, Bondad-Reantaso MG (eds): Diseases in Asian Aquaculture V. AFS-FHS, Manila, 2005, pp 125-136.

6 Subasinghe RP, Arthur JR (eds): Regional Workshop on Preparedness and Response to Aquatic Animal Health Emergencies in Asia. FAO Fisheries Proceedings, FAO, Rome, 2005, no 4.

7 Arthur JR, Baldock FC, Subasinghe RP, McGladdery S: Preparedness and response to aquatic animal health emergencies in Asia: guidelines. FAO Fisheries Technical Paper. FAO, Rome, 2005, no 486.8 Bondad-Reantaso MG, Subasinghe RP: Review of KHV. Aquaculture Asia Pacific Magazine, 2005.

9 Sunarto A, Sumiati T, Hyatt A, Koesharyani I, Antoni R, Itami T: Development of cell line from tail of koi (Cyprinus carpio) and isolation of Koi herpesvirus from Indonesian aquaculture. Book of abstracts from the 6th Symposium on Diseases in Asian Aquaculture, Colombo, 25-28 October 2005.

10 Sunarto A, Rukyani A, Itami T: Indonesian experience on the outbreak of Koi herpesvirus in koi and common carp (Cyprinus carpio). Japan Bull Fish Res Agen 2005;2:15-21.

11 Sunarto A, Cameron A: Response to mass mortality of carp: an Indonesian experiences, in Subasinghe RP, Arthur JR (eds): Regional Workshop on Preparedness and Response to Aquatic Animal Health Emergencies in Asia. FAO Fisheries Proceedings. FAO, Rome, 2005, no 4, pp 87-106.

12 Sunarto A, Cameron A: Epidemiology and control of Koi herpesvirus in Indonesia. Proceedings of the 11th International Symposium on Veterinary Epidemiology and Economics. 2006; (also available at www.sciquest.org.nz)

Dr. Melba B. Reantaso, Department of Fisheries and Aquaculture, Food and Agriculture Organization of the United Nations (FAO), Viale delle Terme di Caracalla, 00100 Rome, Italy
E-mail: Melba.Reantaso@fao.org

Dodet B, the OIE Scientific & Technical Department (eds): The OIE Global Conference on Aquatic Animal Health. Dev Biol (Basel). Basel, Karger, 2007, vol 129, pp 29-34.

Brazilian Aquatic Animal Health Policy

J. Barros Cavalcante Neto, E. de Azevedo Pedrosa Cunha

Ministry of Agriculture, Livestock and Food Supply of Brazil

Key words: aquaculture, Brazil, animal health policy, shrimp production, white spot disease

Abstract: The potential for the development of aquaculture in Brazil is huge. Marine shrimp cultivation in Brazil began in the 1970s and grew rapidly to produce 90,190 tons in 2003. In 2004, several factors including disease, trade disputes, and devaluation of the Real caused the industry to collapse. The appea*rance of white spot disease demonstrated a lack of structure and organisation for responding to the problems involved in managing disease outbreaks. Interaction between the stakeholders involved needs to be organised and facilitated. Dissemination of information and economical stability are necessary for maintaining good practices and the sanitary security of production.

INTRODUCTION

The potential for the development of aquaculture in Brazil is huge. With a total area of 8,511,996 km^2, Brazil is situated in the middle-eastern part of the South American continent and bordered by the Atlantic Ocean. It is divided by the equator in the north with 7% of its area in the Northern hemisphere and 93% in the Southern hemisphere. Ninety-two (92%) of Brazilian territory is located within the Tropics of Cancer and Capricorn. Its intertropical zone shows temperatures throughout the year without significant changes, with an annual mean of 25 to 27°C. The country is bordered by 7,367 km of marine coast, with 5,000,000 hectares of dammed fresh water, approximately 13% of the fresh water available on the planet. It has an extremely favourable climate for the cultivation of aquatic organisms and shows an increasing demand for aquatic products for internal consumption.

Commercial aquaculture in Brazil first started in the 1990s, with around 25,000 tons of aquatic products per year. Since then, several sectors of Brazilian aquaculture such as fish production, crustacean (carcinoculture) and mollusc production have rapidly increased with over 150,000 tons of cultivated aquatic products in 2000. In 2001, that number was estimated at approximately 200,000 t and in 2002 it was nearly 250,000 t.

Marine Shrimp Cultivation

Marine shrimp cultivation in Brazil began in the 1970s, initially with the Farfantepenaeus brasiliensis and Marsupenaeus japonicus species. In the late 1980s, the activity started to show its professional potential and new investments were made based on the introduction of new species of animals (Figure 1).

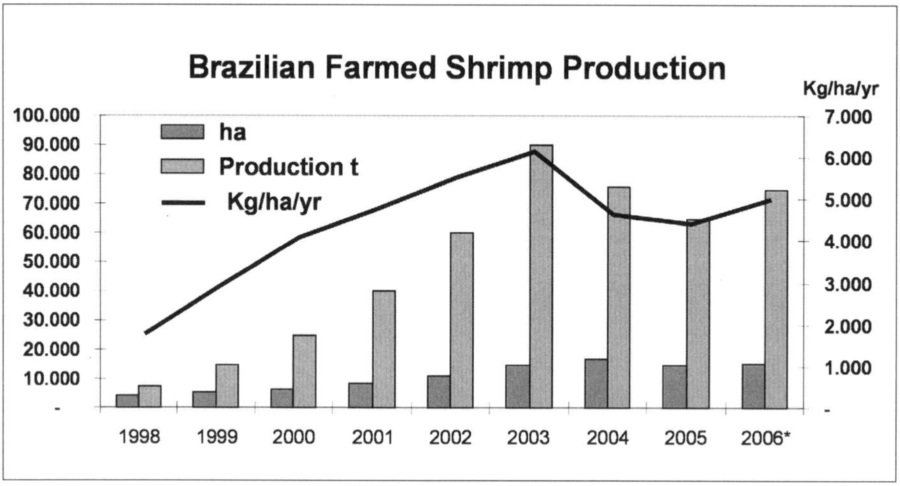

Fig. 1: The Brazilian farmed shrimp production

In 2003, shrimp production was at 90,190 tons. In 2004, however, the industry experienced a 16% decrease with 75,904 tons. There are several reasons for the drop in production: the occurrence of certain diseases; intensive farming methods; and a trade dispute, in which Brazil was accused of dumping, led to a trade ban on Brazilian shrimp. Another factor that contributed to reduced production was the devaluation of the Brazilian currency, the Real, compared to the American dollar. The sum of these factors resulted in the collapse of the sector, which exports 70% of its product.

Today, the Northeastern region, with 90.6% of the total cultivated area, produces 93.1% of Brazil's shrimp, concentrated mostly in the states of Rio Grande do Norte, Ceará and Pernambuco. Commercial farmers own 52.7% of the shrimp production area and they have new technologies and specialized consultants. About 71.4% of all shrimp farmers are considered small producers and they own 15% of the shrimp production area in the country with an average holding area of 3.7 hectares (Figure 2).

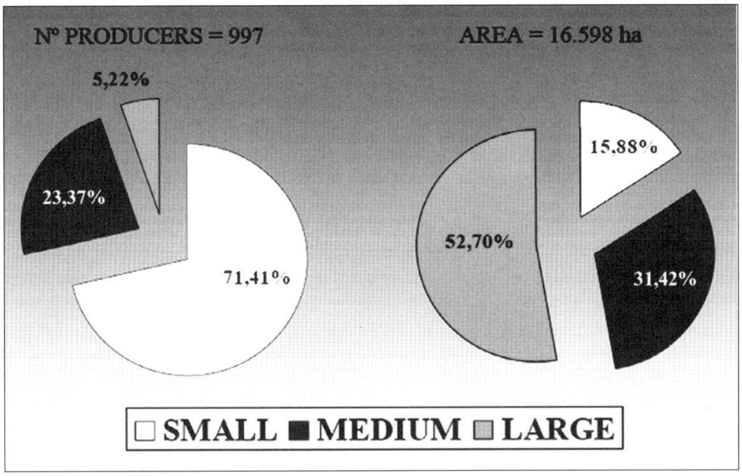

Fig. 2: The Brazilian shrimp farming profile (2005)

The Structure of Brazilian Veterinary Authorities and Controls

The official Veterinarian Service is structured by 3,378 local service offices and 2,378 official veterinarians. The federal instance of the Brazilian Veterinarian Service works mutually with the state instances. The federal instance is responsible for legislating and auditing the state Veterinarian Service, which extends epidemiological surveillance to rural premises. Activities are delegated by formal agreement between the federal and state instances.

The private sector, involved with the public sector, gathers in associations or cooperatives and participates in state or municipal committees and contributes to the decisions taken and to the administration of private funds in case of disease occurrence.

Regulation and the Shrimp Industry

For more than ten years, the importation of Litopenaeus vannamei, an exotic species to Brazil, endangered the country with the possibility of introduction of diseases, despite the surveillance and restrictions imposed by the official veterinarian and environmental authorities. Concerns raised by the increase in shrimp production activity and the notification of diseases in other countries led the Brazilian Veterinarian Authorities to impose, by legislation, restrictions on the importation of crustaceans and crustacean derived products in 1999.

In 2002, the Brazilian Ministry of Agriculture, Livestock and Food Supply started to form the National Program on Aquatic Animal Health which was brought into legislation in July, 2003, after the publication of the Normative Instruction nº 53. In 2003, the federal government also created the Fisheries and Aquaculture Secretariat which is responsible for supporting the Brazilian aquaculture agribusiness. Specific areas of support include helping farmers organize, and industrialisation of production.

Today, the entities involved in aquaculture regulation are working on regulatory norms and on the organisation of the aquatic animal production chain with emphasis on capacity building with respect to official veterinarians.

White Spot Disease in Brazil

The first report of white spot disease in Brazil was confirmed in January, 2005, in the state of Santa Catarina. In August of the same year, the disease was also diagnosed in the state of Ceará (Figure 3). The outbreaks in Santa Catarina occurred in the Imaruí municipality in three premises with a total population of 18,500,000 animals. Clinical signs of the disease were registered and the mortality varied from 50% to 95%. In the municipality of Aracati, in the state of Ceará, the disease occurred on a farm with a total population of 5,000,000 animals with clinical signs; mortality was estimated at 40%. Measures to prevent the spread of the disease were taken and surveillance was reinforced, mostly in reproductive and larvae establishments, where the shrimp production chain begins.

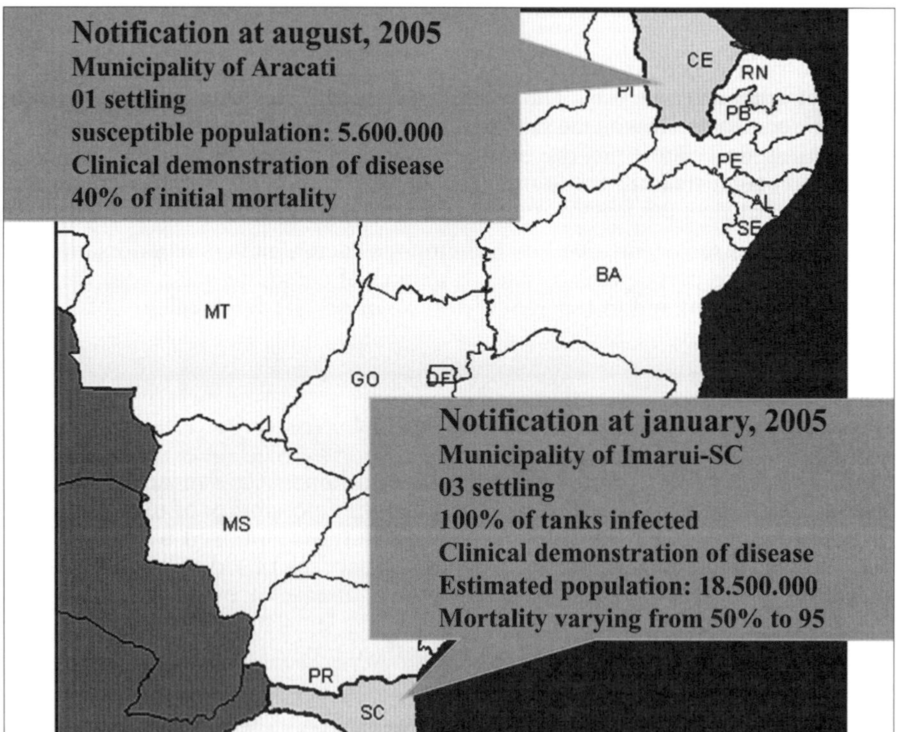

Fig. 3: The 2005 white spot disease outbreak in Brazil

The lack of private funds for reimbursement after the adoption of sanitary measures has aggravated the difficulties involved in the investigation and contributed to the economic collapse of thc farmcrs involved. Due to the weather, economic issues and the lack of experience in facing a disease such as white spot disease, production in these premises has been interrupted. Fear of the economic losses caused by the disease has caused some farmers to try to get environmental licenses for tilapia production, in order to diversify their activity, or to quit shrimp production altogether. The farmers involved in the disease episodes have not yet been able to overcome the losses.

Discussion

The appearance of white spot disease demonstrated a lack of structure and organisation for responding to the problems involved in managing disease outbreaks. For example, the sanitary measures that were taken were hampered by the occurrence of heavy rains because long periods of sun were needed for the full drainage and complete disinfection of the breeding tanks. In addition, it is particularly difficult to set a monitoring standard in Brazil because of the variation in climate throughout the country, the great extent and geographical conformation of the country, as well as different types of technologies adopted on different premises. Since the carcinoculture sector is a new production system in Brazil, there is a lack of veterinarians trained in aquatic pathology. Few veterinarian medical schools in the country are prepared to teach aquatic animal pathology. Finally, the sector has undergone intensification of production, with over 120 shrimp per m^2, without assessment of the impact of these practices on the production areas and the environment and without the necessary technological support. This compromises production conditions and increases vulnerability to pathogen proliferation and environmental changes.

The sensitivity of aquatic animals to weather, raising practices and other factors influencing production may disguise disease occurrence. This makes epidemiological surveillance difficult, especially when the official veterinarian service does not monitor continuously and the farmer is not aware of the importance of disease notification for the stability of the production chain. Therefore, the reimbursement fund and sanitary education are essential tools for the official veterinarian services.

Interaction between the stakeholders involved needs to be organised and facilitated for the dissemination of information and promoting the economical stability necessary for maintaining good practices and the sanitary security of production activity. The interface of aquaculture regulatory organs is not an easy task and needs to be harmonised by legislation and actions. Scientific knowledge and publications need to be made available to the official services. Research on animal species, diseases and the production capacity of cultivated areas can inform with techniques that have less environmental impact and the identification of the most adequate species to be raised in one area. This must not only be a worry of the farmers, but also a concern for regulatory organs.

We need a perfect interface among OIE Reference Laboratories and Veterinarian Services, so that diagnoses made for private interests, often without knowledge of the country of origin of the animals, are notified to the official veterinary service of that country and then to the OIE.

Dr. Eduardo de Azevedo Pedrosa Cunha, Ministério da Agricultura, Pecuária e Abastecimento, Esplanada dos Ministerius, Bloco D, CEP 70043 Brasilia DF
E-mail: eduardocunha@agricultura.gov.br

Dodet B, the OIE Scientific & Technical Department (eds): The OIE Global Conference on Aquatic Animal Health. Dev Biol (Basel). Basel, Karger, 2007,vol 129, pp 35-40.

Contribution of Science to Farm-Level Aquatic Animal Health Management

F. Corsin[1], G. Giorgetti[2], C.V. Mohan[1]

[1] Network of Aquaculture Centres in Asia-Pacific (NACA), Suraswadi Building, Department of Fisheries, Kasetsart University Campus, Ladyao, Jatujak, Bangkok 10900, Thailand

[2] Istituto Zooprofilattico Sperimentale dell'Abruzzo e del Molise 'G.Caporale', via Campo Boario, 64100 Teramo, Italy

Key words: science-based management, aquatic animal health, better management practices, Asia

Abstract: The contribution of science to farm level disease management is a story of two worlds. The development of effective vaccines has allowed for the control of important salmonid diseases such as furunculosis, yersiniosis and vibriosis and has significantly reduced farmers' reliance on antibiotics. Control of diseases for which cost-effective vaccines have yet to be developed has been achieved through the development of increasingly targeted antibiotics and chemotherapeutants. Increasingly, accurate and rapid diagnostic and water quality tests have allowed farmers to improve farm-level aquatic animal health management. In developed countries, these achievements have been possible thanks to the strong link between science and farm management. This link has been assisted by the presence of strong farmer organizations capable of coordinating research projects and hosting meetings at which scientific information is discussed and disseminated.

Although Asia is responsible for the production of about 90% of aquaculture products, it presents a rather different picture from the above. Science has indeed made significant progress in health management but the links with farm management are still weak. Management practices capable of preventing important health problems in shrimp and fish farming are still poorly adopted by farmers. This is largely due to constraints in the dissemination of information to the large number of producers involved, the limited resources of both producers and their countries and the lack of effective farmer organizations capable of liaising with the scientific world. Recently, the Asian region has witnessed some successful examples of aquatic animal health management through the adoption of simple Better Management Practices. Efforts so far have been largely focused on shrimp farming, although activities have been initiated to adopt a similar approach to other commodities. The need for both observational and experimental epidemiological studies to identify simple and affordable farm practices for the control of aquatic animal diseases is highlighted.

Introduction

In response to the rapid growth of the aquaculture sector both in terms of production and value and to the increasing diversification of aquaculture commodities being produced, increasing efforts have been devoted by scientists towards the investigation of aquatic animal health (AAH) issues. These efforts have been focused on several aspects of AAH management, although arguably most often they ultimately targeted the development of strategies that may be adopted by producers to control aquatic animal diseases, such as the use of a chemical, drug or vaccine, the adoption of a certain diagnostic procedure, the farming of a specific pathogen resistant species or family, etc. However, the extent to which scientific research has actually contributed to the development and uptake of farm-level aquatic animal health management has yet to be fully understood.

This manuscript aims at exploring the role played by science in responding to important aquatic animal diseases and providing information on whether research findings have been effectively converted into farm-level management practices.

Identifying Needs For Aquatic Animal Health Management

In order to assess if science has contributed to farm level AAH management, it is necessary to first identify the needs to be addressed. Needs may be examined by looking at the most important aquaculture commodities and determining whether those commodities are affected by important diseases.

The importance of different aquaculture commodities can be measured in several ways; total production in terms of quantity and value is the most common measurement. The Food and Agriculture Organization (FAO) provides annual country-level data on both the quantity and value of aquaculture [1]. Averaging species-level data from 1990 up to the last available data point on the FAO database (i.e. 2004) would allow for the identification of important commodities, minimising the effect of short-lived events. This method shows that major commodities in terms of quantity appear to be bivalves and carps (ranking 1-8), with tilapia and Atlantic salmon ranking 9th and 10th, respectively (Table 1). In terms of value, the first place is occupied by giant tiger shrimp (*Penaeus monodon*), with bivalves and carps still playing an important role, followed by salmonids (Atlantic salmon and rainbow trout occupying the 6th and 11th position respectively) and white-leg shrimp (*Penaeus vannamei*).

The assessment of whether aquaculture commodities of importance are affected by serious diseases can be done by looking at the OIE list of diseases and other information contained in the OIE Aquatic Code and Manual. OIE documents reveal that most of the major commodity groups are affected by OIE listed diseases. Four of the 25 diseases listed in the 2006 Aquatic Code affect the giant tiger shrimp. Bivalves are affected by five OIE listed diseases, two of which also affect Pacific cupped oyster (*Crassostrea gigas*). Carps are also affected by OIE listed diseases, with two affecting common carp (*Cyprinus carpio*). Similarly, OIE listed diseases affect also salmonids, with Atlantic salmon (*Salmo salar*) and rainbow trout (*Oncorhynchus mykiss*) being each susceptible to 3 OIE listed diseases.

Table 1: Ranking of different aquaculture commodities in terms of global production, quantity and value

Rank	Production quantity Species	Average 1990-2004 (million m.t.)	Production Value Species	Average 1990-2004 (billion USD)
1	Pacific cupped oyster	2.999	Giant tiger shrimp	3.419
2	Silver carp	2.883	Pacific cupped oyster	2.771
3	Grass carp	2.554	Silver carp	2.538
4	Common carp	2.183	Common carp	2.459
5	Japanese carpet shell	1.471	Grass carp	2.273
6	Bighead carp	1.377	Atlantic salmon	2.183
7	Yesso scallop	0.969	Japanese carpet shell	1.799
8	Crucian carp	0.940	White-leg shrimp	1.445
9	Nile tilapia	0.756	Yesso scallop	1.327
10	Atlantic salmon	0.664	Bighead carp	1.237

Assessing Whether Science Addresses Needs

The information presented above indicates that carps, bivalves and giant tiger shrimp are species of major importance in terms of production, quantity and value. Salmonids are also important, especially in terms of value, although they do not rank at the very top. These commodities are all susceptible to important diseases. Efforts should therefore be devoted to the study of diseases affecting these commodities, perhaps with a slight bias towards carps, bivalves and giant tiger shrimp.

However, a search of the Aquatic Sciences and Fisheries Abstracts (ASFA) database conducted in October, 2006, on publications issued from 1990 onwards, indicated that salmonids consistently received the most research attention. A total of 2,287 and 2,283 abstracts corresponded to queries on "salmon and health" and "trout and health", respectively. On the contrary, "carps and health" generated only 885 hits, with "common carps and health" leading to less than 300 abstracts. Similarly, "bivalve and health" and "tiger shrimp/prawn and health" identified only 576 and 101 publications, respectively.

Understanding Biases

To understand the reasons why a greater deal of effort is being devoted to the study of health problems in salmonids in spite of their relatively lower importance in terms of quantity and value, it is important to explore differences between different aquaculture commodities.

It is possible that the limited research conducted on bivalve diseases is due to the difficulties in controlling health problems in animals that are generally grown in open water, feed on natural food and do not have an adaptive immune system. Although the latter would also be applicable to crustaceans, these arguments do not seem to explain the differences observed in the amount of research input devoted to salmonid health, when compared to cyprinids or shrimp.

A rapid examination of these commodities indicates that Atlantic salmon is produced in 14 countries of which, according to FAO data [1], the most important are Norway, Chile, the United Kingdom, Canada, the Faeroe Islands and the USA and with production primarily dominated by large companies. Rainbow trout farming is conducted in 59 countries, among which Chile, Norway, Denmark and other European countries dominate. Production is most commonly conducted under intensive conditions and by relatively better-off farmers. Farming of salmonids is also conducted for recreational purposes.

When looking at the production systems for carps and shrimp, a different picture emerges. More than two-thirds of common carp is produced in China and most other important producing countries (e.g. India, Indonesia, etc.) are also located in Asia. Production is dominated by a very large number of small-scale, often poor, producers. Giant tiger shrimp production is also largely conducted in Asian developing countries such as Vietnam, Indonesia and India by millions of poorer small-scale farmers.

There are other important differences in the production of the above commodities. Salmonid aquaculture, and the aquaculture sector in general, in developed countries show a high degree of organization when compared with cyprinid or shrimp farming. Although arguably biased towards resource-rich institutions, the Aquaculture Network Information Centre (AquaNIC) lists 195 aquaculture organisations, only six of which are located in Asia and not one of which is a farmer organization. Producers' organizations play a critical role in identifying and addressing research needs. The Federation of European Aquaculture Producers (FEAP) is a classical example of a successful producers' organization. FEAP is composed of 28 associations spanning across 23 countries. Its members are responsible for the production of 1.2 million tonnes of aquaculture products for a value exceeding three billion Euros [2]. FEAP supports the designing and implementation of research projects, holds conferences with sessions on fish diseases, disseminates fish health information to its members on a regular basis, develops Codes of Conduct for the sector and issues resolutions which present producers' views on AAH matters to governmental institutions.

Carps and shrimp producers, like farmers of many other aquaculture commodities in Asia, face several constraints to properly benefiting from the contribution of science to AAH management. The resources of Asian farmers are often too limited to properly address their needs. They are often too poor to implement the recommended AAH management practices or to support research, unless they are ised and express their needs or to accumulate funds to support research efforts. In addition, they are often too numerous to be reached by scientific findings through the available extension systems.

A Story of Two Worlds

The contribution of science to AAH disease management therefore appears to be a story of two worlds. The development of effective vaccines has allowed for the control of important salmonid diseases such as furunculosis and vibriosis and has significantly reduced farmers' reliance on antibiotics. Control of diseases for which cost-effective vaccines have yet to be developed has been achieved through the development of increasingly targeted antibiotics and chemotherapeutants. Increasingly, accurate and rapid diagnostic and water quality tests, sometimes incorporated into data-loggers, have allowed farmers to improve farm-level AAH management. In developed countries, these achievements have been possible thanks to the strong link between science and farm management. This link has been assisted by the presence of strong farmers' organizations capable of coordinating research projects and hosting meetings at which scientific information is discussed and disseminated.

Although Asia is responsible for the production of about 90% of the world's aquaculture products, it presents a rather different picture. Science has indeed made significant progress in AAH management but the links with farm management are still weak. Management practices for preventing important health problems in shrimp and fish are still poorly adopted by farmers. This is largely due to constraints in disseminating information to the large number of producers involved, to the limited resources of both producers and their countries and to the lack of effective farmer organizations capable of liaising with the scientific world. The lack of organization and limited resources of producers has also limited efforts towards the development of vaccines for diseases that are important to Asian producers.

Bridging the Gap

The news is not all bad. Recently, the Asian region has witnessed some successful examples of AAH management by small-scale producers through the adoption of Better Management Practices (BMP). BMP are simple, cost-effective and system-specific management practices which address AAH management broadly, also targeting food safety and environmental and socio-economic sustainability. BMP are generally developed using available scientific knowledge and epidemiological (i.e. population-based) studies that identify key issues that need to be addressed. BMP are then disseminated to farming communities who play an active role in their pilot testing. Efforts to address the sustainability of the shrimp farming sector in a wide range of Asian countries have shown outstanding results. BMP designed to convert the International Principles for Responsible Shrimp Farming [3] into practice have been developed and implemented by small-scale producers in India, Vietnam and other countries, leading to increased profits and improved product quality [4,5]. Similar efforts are now underway for the production of other aquaculture commodities that are important to Asian producers such as cyprinids and marine fish [6].

Conclusions

Science can contribute to farm-level aquatic animal health management. Experiences from the aquaculture sector of developed countries have clearly shown how allocation of resources to research, the creation of producers' organizations and two-way communication between scientists and farmers has led to the successful development of the sector.

The challenges faced by the Asian aquaculture sector are still too many to allow producers to effectively benefit from research efforts. Nevertheless, the recent adoption of innovative approaches, such as the development and implementation of Better Management Practices, represent a promising way forward. Government and the private sector alike are increasingly pursuing such innovative approaches, targeting not only the management of AAH problems, but also the overall sustainability of the aquaculture sector.

References

1 FAO FISHSTAT Plus: FAO Fisheries Department, Fishery Information, Data and Statistics Unit). Aquaculture production: quantities 1950-2004 and Aquaculture production: values 1984-2004. FISHSTAT Plus: Universal software for fishery statistical time series. Version 2.3. 2000. Food and Agriculture Organization of the United Nations, 2006.

2 The Federation of European Aquaculture Producers (FEAP): www.feap.info/feap

3 FAO/NACA/UNEP/WB/WWF: International Principles for Responsible Shrimp Farming. Network of Aquaculture Centres in Asia-Pacific (NACA). Bangkok, Thailand, 2006, 20pp.

4 Corsin F, Mohan CV, Padiyar PA, Yamamoto K, Chanratchakool P, Phillips MJ: Codes of practice and better management: a solution for shrimp health management?, in Reantaso MB, Mohan CV, Crumlish M and Subasinghe R (eds.): Diseases in Asian Aquaculture 6. Fish Health Section, Asian Fisheries Society, in press.

5 Padiyar PA, Phillips MJ, Bhat BV, Mohan CV, Ravi BG, Mohan ABC, Sai P: Cluster level adoption of Better Management Practices in shrimp (*P. monodon*) farming: an experience from Andhra Pradesh, India, in Reantaso MB, Mohan CV, Crumlish M and Subasinghe R (eds.). Diseases in Asian Aquaculture 6. Fish Health Section, Asian Fisheries Society, in press.

6 MOFI/World Bank: Guidelines for environmental management of aquaculture investments in Vietnam. Technical Note N.37564. The World Bank, Washington, USA, 2006.

Dr. Flavio Corsin, Network of Aquaculture Centres in Asia-Pacific (NACA), Suraswadi Building, Department of Fisheries, Kasetsart University Campus, Ladyao, Jatujak, Bangkok 10900, Thailand.
E-mail: flavio.corsin@gmail.com

Dodet B, the OIE Scientific & Technical Department (eds): The OIE Global Conference on Aquatic Animal Health. Dev Biol (Basel). Basel, Karger, 2007,vol 129, pp 41-51.

Modelling for Disease Preparedness and Response

A.G. Murray, R.S. Raynard

Fisheries Research Services Marine Laboratory, Aberdeen, UK

Key words: modelling, epidemiological models, risk analysis, disease management

Abstract: Modelling is a useful tool for the understanding and hence, potentially, control of disease. In an emergency situation, obtaining data to validate detailed models may be difficult. However, modelling can be useful in aiding the management of disease, if the objectives are not too ambitious. For example, import risk analysis can use models to minimise the risk of outbreaks. Modelling can also be used to maximise the power of surveillance data to ensure that any outbreak is detected as rapidly as possible. Methods of modelling spread of disease, and measures to prevent this, including SIR-style epidemiological models, models of disease control zones and contact network models can be used to identify and minimise the potential scale of an epidemic. Finally, economic and ecological models can be used to assess the impact of outbreaks. A range of simple models is likely to be of more use than a single comprehensive model.

INTRODUCTION

Models describe the interactions in a system using a simplified form that gives insight into the system's behaviour. Here the use of mathematical models to devise strategies to prevent or control disease outbreaks is described. Such mathematical models may be devised empirically, with an outcome variable fitted as a function of other observed variables, without explanation of the system's behaviour. Alternatively, models may be devised conceptually, with the modeller's understanding of the system's behaviour described in terms of equations and the solutions compared with observations. Conceptual models can produce more insight into a system's behaviour, but validation may be difficult.

Data is required to build and validate models. Obtaining sufficient data during a disease outbreak is difficult, and so results are likely to be uncertain. Therefore, for aquatic disease emergencies, simple, robust, models used to provide advice to managers are likely to be of more use than detailed models used to drive a control policy.

In this paper, modelling approaches that may be useful in helping managers to avoid outbreaks, or to minimise their impact should they occur, are briefly described. The models are divided into those concerning risk of introduction, those for evaluating the power of sampling regimes for the detection of an outbreak, models of disease spread within an area, and models of consequences of an outbreak.

Materials and Methods

Models to reduce the risk of disease introduction

Modelling of introduction risk for exotic aquatic diseases is relatively well understood (relative to other aspects of aquatic disease control) in terms of the release assessment phase of Import Risk Analysis [1]. In practice, many Import Risk Assessments consist largely of this phase, and there has been particularly little emphasis on consequence assessment.

The release assessment involves one or more chains of events which are followed to produce a probability of the pathogen being transported from a source country into the receiving country (Fig. 1). The more detail that can be included (and validated) in such models the more clearly the principle risk factors can be identified and consequences of modification assessed. Models can be qualitative, identifying risks as high, low, negligible etc., or they can be quantitative (e.g. 0.1% year-1). Monte-Carlo methods may be used to assess overall risk within the confidence ranges around individual risk parameters using different distribution patterns (e.g. uniform or triangular), especially for complex networks. Data to support such models can come from many sources, including expert opinion, if more objective data (e.g. movement records or efficacy of laboratory disinfection) is unavailable.

Models for rapid detection

The more rapidly an exotic pathogen is detected the less time it has to spread. Interpretation of samples is based on a model that ranges from assumption of 100% specificity and sensitivity for 10% prevalence in a single uniformly mixed population (the traditional 30 fish sample), to risk based surveillance [2] which is based on sophisticated assumptions of risk that a site may become infected and risk of transmission should a site become infected.

Sampling models should take into account sensitivity and specificity of tests, including combinations of tests, to achieve acceptable levels of false positive and false negatives. Simple models can calculate the proportion of false positive values using positive predictive power.

$$PPV = SeP/(SeP + (1 - Sp)(1 - P))$$

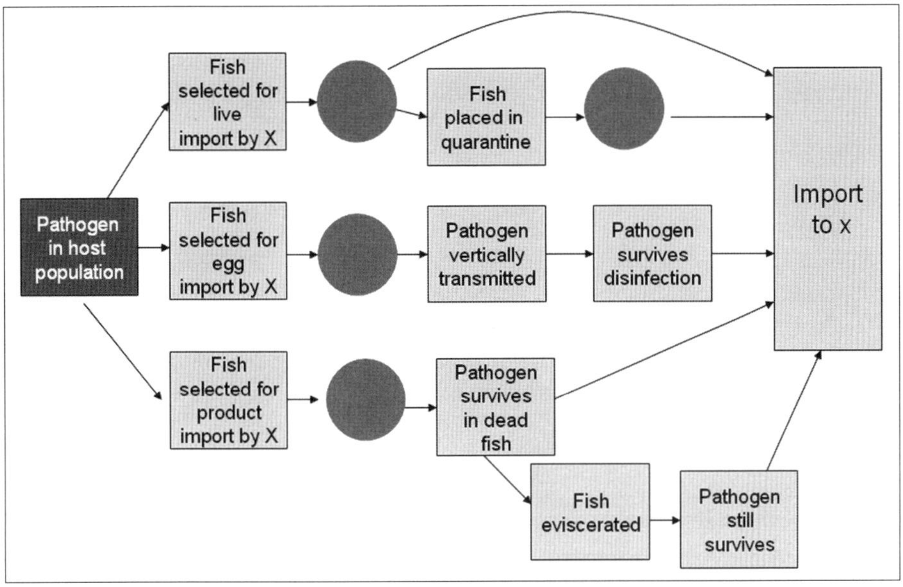

Fig. 1: A simple model for the analysis of a fish pathogen being imported to country X. Black circles represent opportunities for surveillance when a pathogen may be detected. Other boxes are labelled. Flow probabilities through each pathway connecting the source with country X are the product of probability of each step in the pathway, and these pathway probabilities are summed for all pathways.

Estimates of P are Baysian and as these change so does the estimate of power of a positive result, leading to further changes in estimates of P [2]; thus understanding the true power of surveillance can require sophisticated modelling. Multiple testing methods may be used within a country including passive and active surveillance methods, and total available information on a country's disease status incorporates both.

A method of illustrating the power of the detection methods available is the scenario tree under which the process of detection is broken down to reflect different steps in the detection process and in the structure of the problem (Fig. 2). These nodes may be infection nodes (e.g. farm is or is not infected), detection nodes (e.g. inspector visits), category nodes (e.g. freshwater or marine sites) and switch nodes (modelling nodes used to turn off/on different simulated sampling regimes). Nodes are linked so that a chain is required to estimate the probability of detecting disease (e.g. $DD = 1 - \exp(1 - F \times p1 \times p2 \times p3 \times Se)$, where F is the number of farms, p1 is the probability a farm is infected, p2 is the probability an inspector visits it, p3 the probability they take a sample, and Se the sampling sensitivity.

As with risk analysis, parameters used within the model represented by the decision tree may be derived by expert opinion or by more objective analysis of data. Sensitivity and specificity can be evaluated by laboratory studies, but sampling in the field may require cross comparison of results from different tests. Factors such as frequency of inspection or numbers of farms can be determined from official records. The model structure can be modified to analyse for different assumptions and Monte-Carlo methods can be used to determine how uncertainty in the parameters affects estimated probability of detection.

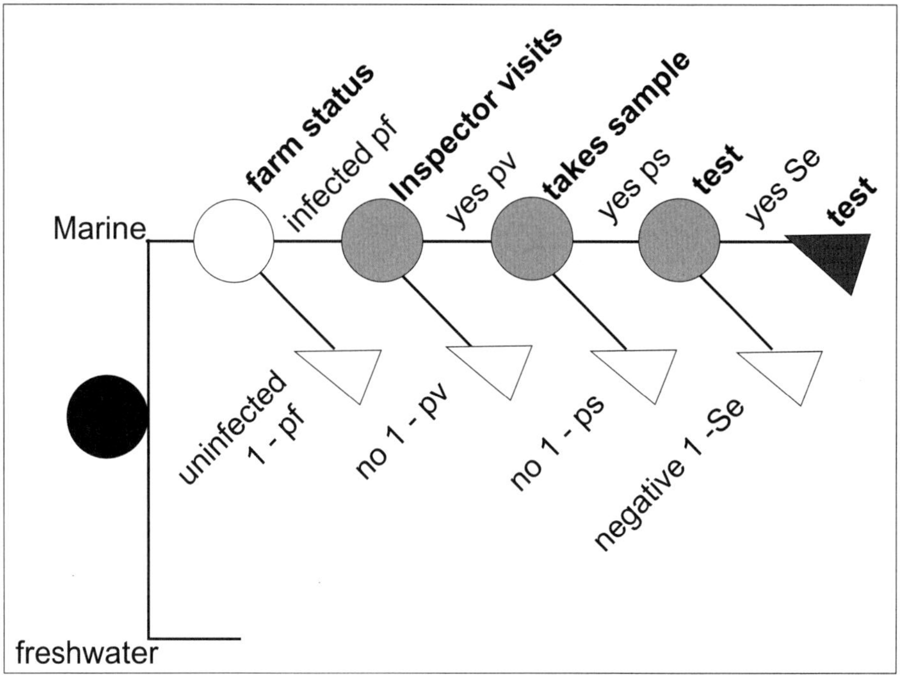

Fig. 2: A simple model of the probability of surveillance detecting a pathogen. For each infected farm the probability is the product of pf × pv × ps × Se. A similar path exists for marine farms, although p values may be different at each step.

Models of spread of disease

There are several different types of model that may be useful for identifying conditions favouring (or inhibiting) disease spread. These include SIR-type epidemic models, hydrodynamic-based models of pathogen transport, and network structure models of movements of fish between farms and other sites.

SIR-type epidemic models

SIR models divide the host population into susceptible (S), infected (I), and removed individuals (R); this last may be dead or recovered and immune. The basic SIR model was developed in 1927 and is of the form:

$$dS/dt = -\beta SI$$
$$dI/dt = \beta SI - \alpha I$$
$$dR/dt = \alpha I$$

Such models have the capacity to describe basic properties of epidemics and have been fitted to many specific cases, including herpesvirus in wild pilchards [3] and sea lice of farmed salmon [4]. More complex models incorporate a more detailed population structure and involve modification of the simple dependence of transmission on population density [5]. The simple population density dependent transmission term, βSI, may be replaced by a variety of different formulae including the population density independent $\beta SI/N$, where $N = S + I + R$. This formula was developed for vector driven diseases but may be useful to describe transmission among schooling fish where school density is independent of the larger scale population density [3].

Model fitting and validation generally requires data derived from observing the spread of an epidemic. Such data are unlikely to be obtainable in the early stage of an emergency, and [4] only become available later.

Hydrodynamic-particle models

Aquatic pathogen transmission may be heavily dependent on the movement of water. Models describing the movement of sea lice [6,7] and infectious salmon anaemia virus (ISAV) [8] have used coupled particle and hydrodynamic models to derive patterns of distribution that may result from pathogens released from a site. A simpler approach is to use tidal excursion distance [7] to determine a radius over which pathogens may disperse:

$$X = UT/\pi$$

A coupling of very simple hydrodynamic and particle decay models [7] has been used to estimate distances over which pathogens may be transported at biologically significant concentrations.

Principles of hydrodynamic modelling are well established [6], although validation of a model for a particular environment may require extensive fieldwork. This data concerns the physical environment and can be obtained in the absence of an epidemic; the models may serve other purposes (e.g. water-quality modelling). Data on pathogen decay can be obtained experimentally [7].

Network modelling

Network models are used to include the non-local spread of disease, for example with the transport of fish between sites on different river systems [9,10]. Models have also been developed from first principles to look at the effect of mixing different degrees of local and long-distance transport [11]. Such models result in assessments of path length between any two sites, and hence how easily disease may be transmitted. Sites do not interact equally. Some sites, e.g., hatcheries, may interact with many others, while isolated on-growing sites may interact only weakly if at all with other sites; the distribution may follow a power-law [9]. Data on numbers and patterns of interactions can be obtained from inspector's movement records. A simplified model is used in this paper to illustrate networks. In this model 300 sites are arranged in a ring and, if infected, have a probability in each model time step of spreading the infection to either a neighbouring site or to a randomly selected site anywhere in the ring. By manipulating the probability of long-distance transmission, its influence on the speed with which infection spreads through the farms is illustrated.

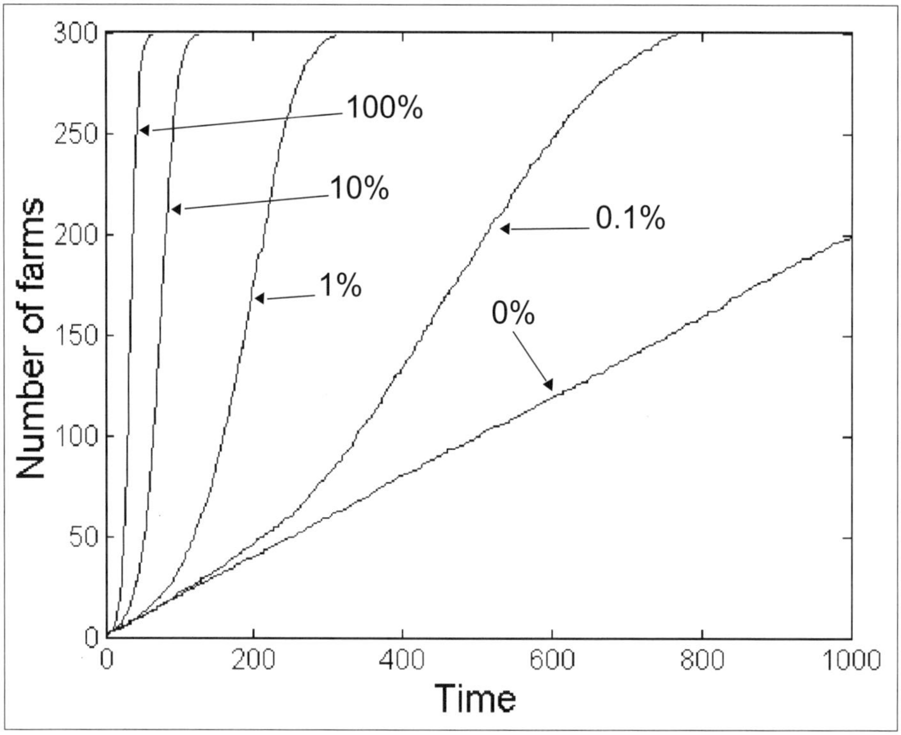

Fig.3: The median number of sites infected versus time for a ring of 300 sites that interact with immediate neighbours or randomly throughout the ring at the probability indicated on the graph lines. Even a very small number of non-local interactions greatly reduce the time for infection to spread throughout the ring (e.g. 1% of such exchanges leads to an 80% reduction in time).

Modelling the impact of disease

Economic modelling can be used to assess likely costs of disease, should an outbreak occur. This involves estimating fish mortality and value, which depends on the age at which they are lost, with salvageable sale value and reduced production costs removed. A budget model has been derived for cardiomyopathy syndrome including direct losses, reduced costs and salvageable value of culled fish [12]. It is with such endemic pathogens that reliable modelling can be carried out, while the scale of impact of novel diseases, and their costs and control are difficult to evaluate.

Models can be used to predict the impact of disease using observations of the prevalence of symptoms. This method has been used to assess the impact of the fungal parasite *Icthyophonus* on herring stocks available for fisheries [13].

Ecological modelling methods can be used to examine the indirect effects of disease on other species and the interaction of disease with fishing activity. Such models treat disease as a predator competing for fish stocks with other predators or fishermen.

RESULTS

Models to reduce the risk of disease introduction

The release assessment of import risk analysis has been developed quite effectively to become a respected tool for disease control in the context of freer trade [1]. Obtaining adequate data for the estimation and verification of parameters may be difficult, but the approach is transparent and so provides an effective method for exploring uncertainty. The result of an import assessment model is an estimate of the probability of an import occurring during a given period, preferably with specified uncertainties in that estimate, and insight into ways of reducing this probability, if cost-effective ways exist.

Models for rapid detection

Sampling theory is also quite well-developed and is useful for designing data collection methods for determining a country's disease-free status. Large amounts of data are formally and informally collected and combining this data in a formal transparent way, including the use of scenario trees to make the model visual, can greatly increase confidence in disease free status.

Sampling involves a model of the distribution of infection depending on the aim of the surveillance. Determining disease-free status or prevalence at country level could involve the widespread taking of small samples, for example, which may be too small to determine the infection status of individual rivers or farms, or even fish, when parts of an animal are sampled.

Targeted surveillance leads to more efficient sampling and more rapid detection of infection [2]. More frequent sampling of high risk populations is more likely to detect infection more rapidly than is random sampling. However, targeting requires a model of risk and may weaken the power of surveillance if this model is not adequate.

Modelling is an effective tool for analysing the conditional probabilities of false positive and false negatives under different sampling regimes. At low prevalence high specificity is required, while at high prevalence high sensitivity is required to avoid unmanageable false results. Such modelling can be used to assess the effects of mixing different tests and assuming that the tests are unrelated.

Models of spread of disease

SIR-type epidemiological models

Dynamic models can provide deep insight into the spread of disease. However, the validation of detailed models can require a great deal of data. While such models are useful in later analysis of epidemics [3] or endemic pathogens [4] they may not be practicable for the simulation of specific outbreaks unless experience can be gained from outbreaks that occurred earlier or elsewhere. Simpler models can be used to more rapidly obtain insight into the basic dynamics of epidemics [3]. For example, population density thresholds required for epidemics to occur can be derived from such simple models [5] with different basic assumptions regarding transmission, but not with density independent transmission. Such models show, in general terms, how diseases are likely to be made worse by the side effects of aquaculture, such as higher rates of contact and higher population density leading to an increase in transmission parameter β. The general effects of management actions such as movement restrictions or culling can also be evaluated for given assumptions, including indirect effects through changes in infection pressure.

Hydrodynamic models

Simple tidal excursion models have been used to derive surveillance zones to support a successful ISAV eradication policy in Scotland [7]. Simple coupled hydrodynamic-particle tracking models indicated that this worked because free ISAV were labile and more robust pathogens might be transported beyond the tidal excursion zones [7]. Small control zones were not effective in controlling ISAV in Canada and were shown to be smaller than the scales of tidal mixing determined by hydrodynamic models [8]. Such models are thus demonstrably useful for developing or testing control policies. Risk to wild fish from lice from British Columbian salmon farms, as determined by models, depends on whether the larvae accumulate locally [14] or are transported out to sea [6], which is essentially a hydrodynamic problem.

Network modelling

Theoretical network modelling has been used to show the relative power of transmission randomly throughout a spatial system relative to exchange between neighbours. A surprisingly small number of non-local contacts are required to create a small-world situation in which there is only a short path-length between any two nodes (which might be fish farms) and which greatly accelerates epidemic spread [11]. This principle is illustrated by looking at the spread of disease in a ring of 300 nodes (farms) ranging from transmission between immediate neighbours to purely random transmission, with cases where 10%, 1% or 0.1% of transmission is random. It can be seen that small numbers of random exchanges substantially increase rate of spread (Fig. 3). The implication of this for the management of epidemics is profound; since even a small number of long-distance movements can greatly expand the number of cases in an epidemic, imports may expose countries to high risk of exotic disease.

Network modelling has been developed and tested based on recorded live freshwater fish movements in England [9] and using mean field models based on an asymmetric contact network [10]. Such models are useful for illustrating the potential extent and rapidity of spread of disease in such networks, although it may be less useful than for symmetric networks [10]. Simulated spread in the English contact structure model was usually found to be quite limited, but some outbreaks were very large, reflecting the power law distribution of numbers of movements of fish from different river systems [9].

Modelling impact of disease

The impact of slow-killing diseases such as *Icthyophonus* may be predictable from looking at the current prevalence of symptoms and a simple model relating them to later mortality [13]. Post-epidemic assessment of change in fish stocks, based on models used to assess fish stocks can be used to assess the impact of large epidemics on wild fish. The impact on wild populations may depend on the stage affected and so may recovery following an epidemic [3]. Modelling has the potential to illustrate the financial impact of losses to aquaculture, beyond the crude proportion of the population killed, for example, by looking at the age at which mortality occurs in the light of production costs [12]. Impact assessment is explicitly part of risk and consequence assessment, but it is rarely undertaken in detail.

Mortality can also affect predators, prey or competitors and interact with fisheries. Modelling indirect impact through ecosystems should be possible using ecosystem modelling; some work has been done for pisciverous birds. Fisheries have the potential to interact in quite complex ways with epidemics, with pre-epidemic fishing leading to reduced mortality, provided that disease transmission is related to population density.

Discussion

Modelling may be seen as a useful tool, or rather set of tools, for the management of disease emergencies, provided that the expectations are reasonable. These tools aid in the prevention of disease introduction and the rapid detection, and limitation of spread and consequences should an outbreak occur.

Import risk relates to the release assessment phase of import risk analysis. It is carried out by developing a conceptual series of pathways by which import might occur and then attempting to evaluate the probabilities (and uncertainties around these) associated with each step on the pathways to generate an assessment of the risk of import. This method is fairly well established [1] and allows for transparent discussion of uncertainties surrounding each step in generating the overall risk, and their potential for reduction. It is also a useful means of incorporating data from a variety of sources, including expert opinion.

Rapid detection depends on efficient surveillance. Surveillance is based on the implicit application of models, however, the underlying assumptions of the model must be considered. Specifically, a 30 fish sample is often considered to be the way to ensure a site is free of pathogen. This is appropriate for the detection of epidemic outbreaks, but may fail to detect carrier infection at low prevalence. Similarly, large-scale surveillance for low-prevalence pathogens is quite likely (low probability, but high conditional probability) to produce false-positives even if confirmatory tests are required.

Several approaches are applicable to modelling disease spread, including SIR-type, hydrodynamic, and network models. No one model is likely to describe all aspects of spread [4]. All show great sensitivity with regard to the extent and rapidity of spread of epidemics and the exact nature of transmission between sites or individuals, which is likely to depend on the structure of the industry, the environment, the fish populations and the pathogen itself. If transmission is localised, the potential to bring the epidemic under control is greatly enhanced. Hydrodynamic modelling has proven useful for devising local control zones [7]. Conversely, rare long distance transmission may play a disproportionate role in epidemic spread; most such movements are anthropogenic and so, in principle, controllable. The application of simple versions of these models is a useful step, but obtaining the data for specific pathogens in specific industry structures may be more difficult.

Finally, while consequence modelling is only just beginning to develop, and requires more collaboration with fisheries scientists, ecologists and economists, some practicable tools exist [12,13].

Conclusion

Modelling provides managers with tools, and not with 'answers' (especially in the short-term). Modelling may be applied (e.g. to sampling programmes), without an understanding of the model, or even that a model is being used, leading to the incorrect interpretation of observations. Therefore explicit modelling techniques, which allow individual steps and parameters to be discussed and disputed, can make the assumptions behind epidemic management more transparent. The level of application of modelling to different areas of prevention and control of epidemics is highly variable, with the best established models being simple risk models in the release phase of import risk assessment, and the least consequence assessment of disease outbreaks. In practice, simple models have proven most useful in the control of specific emergencies. However, the more (testable) detail it can incorporate, the more a model can reveal of a system's underlying dynamics.

Acknowledgements

We thank the OIE for funding Dr. Murray's attendance at the Global Conference on Aquatic Animal Health.

References

1 Rodger CJ: Risk analysis in aquatic animal health. Paris, World Organisation for Animal Health, 2001, pp 346.

2 Stark KDC, Regula, G, Hernandez, J, Knopf, L, Fuchs, K, Morris, RS, Davis P: Concepts for risk-based surveillance in the field of veterinary medicine and veterinary public health: Review of current approaches. BMC Health Services Res 2006;6: 1-8.

3 Murray AG, O'Callaghan, M: The numerical and computing methods used to implement models of the spread and impact a major epidemic disease: pilchard herpesvirus, Australia 1995 and 1998/9. Environm Modell Software 2005;20:575-85.

4 Revie CW, Robbins, C, Gettinby, G, Kelly, L, Treasurer JW: A mathematical model of the growth of sea lice *Lepeophtherius salmonis* populations on farmed Atlantic salmon, *Salmo salar* L., in Scotland and its use in the assessment of treatment strategies. J Fish Dis 2005; 28, 603-13.

5 McCallum H, Barlow N, Hone J: How should pathogen transmission be modelled? Trends Ecol Evol 2001;16: 295-300.

6 Brooks KM: The effects of water temperature, salinity, and currents on the survival and distribution of the infective copepodid stage of sea lice (*Lepeophtheirus salmonis*) originating on Atlantic salmon farms in the Broughton Archipelago of British Columbia, Canada. Rev Fish Sci 2005;13:177-204.

7 Murray, AG, Amundrud TL, Gillibrand PA: Models of hydrodynamic pathogen dispersal affecting Scottish salmon production: Modelling shows how Scotland eradicated ISA, but not IPN. Bull Aquacult Assoc Can 2006;105-1: 80-87.

8 Chang BD, Page HF, Losier RJ, Greenberg DA, Chaffey JD, McCurdy EP: Application of a tidal circulation model for fish health management of salmon farms in the Grand Manan Island area, Bay of Fundy. Bull Aquacult Assoc Can 2006;105-1:22-33.

9 Thrush M, Peeler E: Stochastic simulation of live fish movements in England and Wales to predict potential spread of exotic pathogens. Dis Aquat Org 2006;72:115-23.

10 Sharkey KJ, Fernandez C, Morgan KL, Peeler E, Thrush M, Turnbull JF, Bowers RG: Pair-level approximations to the spatio-temporal dynamics of epidemics on asymmetric contact networks. J Math Biol 2006;53:61-85.

11 Watts DJ, Strogatz SH: The collective dynamics of 'small-world' networks. Nature 1998;393:440-442.

12 Brun E, Poppe T, Skrudland A, Jarp J: Cardiomyopathy syndrome in farmed Atlantic salmon *Salmo salar*: occurrence and direct financial losses for Norwegian aquaculture. Dis Aquat Org 2003;56:241-47.

13 Patterson KR: Modelling the impact of disease-induced mortality in an exploited population: The outbreak of the fungal parasite *Ichthyophonus hoferi* in the North Sea herring (*Clupea harengus*). Can J Fish Aquat Sci 1996;53:2870-87.

14 Krkosek M, Lewis MA, Volpe JP: Transmission dynamics of parasitic sea lice from farm to wild salmon. Proc Biol Sci 2005; 272:689-96.

Dr. Alexander G Murray, Fisheries Research Services Marine Laboratory, 375 Victoria Road, Aberdeen AB11 9DB, UK
E-mail: murrays@marlab.ac.uk

Dodet B, the OIE Scientific & Technical Department (eds): The OIE Global Conference on Aquatic Animal Health. Dev Biol (Basel). Basel, Karger, 2007,vol 129, p 53.

Session III

Infrastructure for Disease Surveillance and Emergency Response

Chairperson: *D. Lightner,* USA

Dodet B, the OIE Scientific & Technical Department (eds): The OIE Global Conference on Aquatic Animal Health. Dev Biol (Basel). Basel, Karger, 2007, vol 129, pp 55-64.

Structural Arrangements in Australia for Managing Aquatic Animal Disease Emergencies

E.-M. Bernoth

Office of the Chief Veterinary Officer, Australian Government Department of Agriculture, Fisheries and Forestry, Australia

Key words: AQUAPLAN, Australia, aquatic animal disease, management

Abstract: A major pilchard mortality event in Australia in 1995 highlighted the need for a trans-border approach to aquatic animal health, particularly with respect to disease response. Cooperation between industry and government led to the development of AQUAPLAN – Australia's National Strategic Plan for Aquatic Animal Health. Under AQUAPLAN, the coordination of the national technical response to aquatic animal health emergencies was incorporated into the scope of Australia's Consultative Committee on Emergency Animal Disease, a committee chaired by the Australian Chief Veterinary Officer. The operations of this committee are underpinned by *AQUAVETPLAN*, a series of manuals that outline Australia's approach to national disease preparedness and propose the technical response and control strategies to be activated in a national aquatic animal disease emergency. Simulation exercises provide training to respond to aquatic emergency animal disease events. Some of the lessons learned and challenges ahead are discussed below.

INTRODUCTION

The Constitution of the Commonwealth of Australia provides that the Australian government may make laws on quarantine and international animal health matters including disease reporting, export certification and trade negotiations, while Australia's states and territories have sovereign powers in matters affecting their rural industries, including animal disease control within their borders. The Australian government also advises and coordinates national policy, and, in some circumstances, provides financial assistance for national animal disease control programs. State services administer relevant legislation governing livestock identification and movement (within and between states and territories), disease surveillance, diagnosis, reporting and control of notifiable diseases, chemical residues and other programmes.

Following a major pilchard mortality event in 1995, the need for a transborder approach to aquatic animal health, particularly with respect to disease response, was acknowledged. The then Standing Committee on Fisheries and Aquaculture reported to its Ministerial Council that priority should be given to developing a national response mechanism for fisheries and aquaculture emergencies. Subsequently, several comprehensive reviews were formally tabled within Australia. These were critically assessed and recommendations were made regarding Australia's national response to fisheries and aquaculture emergencies; Australia's quarantine policy including aquatic animal quarantine, and quarantine of imported fish and fish products; and management of incursions of pests, weeds and diseases. In 1997, following a Cabinet decision relating to two of the above reports [1,2], the Australian government allocated funds to the then Commonwealth Department of Primary Industries and Energy, now the Australian Department of Agriculture, Fisheries and Forestry (DAFF), to implement the recommendations of both reports. This included funds to develop a comprehensive aquatic animal health plan for Australia and to address management procedures for aquatic animal disease emergencies in particular. The Australian government's response to these reports recognised that *"there should be a national approach [to fish health] jointly developed by the Commonwealth, states and industry that includes quarantine, research and education and public awareness as key components."* The response further noted that *"... it is also important to ensure that our priorities are correct and that the burden of resources is shared equitably among the beneficiaries"* [3].

AQUAPLAN

Cooperation between industry and government led to the development of AQUAPLAN – Australia's National Strategic Plan for Aquatic Animal Health. The first five-year plan *AQUAPLAN 1998–2003* [4] was broadly aimed at maximising the opportunities for, and profitability of, Australian aquaculture and fisheries, through implementation of discrete projects in eight overarching programmes: international linkages; quarantine; surveillance, monitoring and reporting; preparedness and response; awareness; research and development; legislation, policies and jurisdiction; and resources and funding.

The plan's first successor, *AQUAPLAN 2005–2010* [5], was developed to address, on the basis of a performance review of its predecessor [6], specific priority areas within aquatic animal health. It is a broad, comprehensive strategy to further build and enhance capacity for the management of aquatic animal health in Australia.

There are seven main strategies within *AQUAPLAN 2005–2010*. Government and private sectors have identified priority projects under these seven strategies to achieve the plan's objectives. Together, these objectives will help to maximise Australia's ability to control aquatic animal disease outbreaks, maintain market access, support quality assurance, and improve the productivity and sustainability of its aquatic animal production industries. The seven *AQUAPLAN 2005–2010* strategies are as follows: enhanced integration and scope of aquatic animal health surveillance in Australia; harmonisation of approaches to aquatic animal health in Australia; enhancement of aquatic animal emergency disease preparedness and response arrangements; education and training in the aquatic animal health sector; welfare standards for aquaculture; appropriate use of therapeutics for aquatic animal health management; and aquatic animal health management as a part of ecologically sustainable development. Like its predecessor, *AQUAPLAN 2005–2010* was developed by government and private industry sectors under the management of a joint committee. Both plans were designed to link to, or modify, existing arrangements for terrestrial animals, to prevent duplication and make sensible use of limited resources.

A Framework For The Management Of Emergency Animal Disease Events

Australia's national system for preparing for, and responding to, emergency animal disease (EAD) events, including those in aquatic animals, encompasses all activities relating to disease surveillance, monitoring and response. These activities are carried out by the Australian government, state and territory governments, industries, the Commonwealth Scientific and Industrial Research Organisation (CSIRO), private veterinarians and laboratories, and other animal and aquatic animal health workers. As with terrestrial animal disease emergencies, the operational capacity for dealing with aquatic EAD events in each state and territory is managed through each jurisdiction's emergency management committee. This structure brings together a broad range of resources to help fisheries, aquaculture and aquatic animal health authorities deal with any problem.

Consultative Committee on Emergency Animal Disease

Under *AQUAPLAN 1998–2003*, the coordination of the national technical response to aquatic EAD events was incorporated into the scope of Australia's Consultative Committee on Emergency Animal Disease (CCEAD). This advisory committee is made up of the Australian Chief Veterinary Officer (CVO) as chair, representatives from the Australian Quarantine and Inspection Service and Biosecurity Australia (both within DAFF), the CVO (or the director of the fisheries department) from each state and territory government, and the head of the CSIRO Australian Animal Health Laboratory. Technical representatives from industry may also be invited to participate.

The CCEAD's mission is to *"... coordinate the national technical response to terrestrial and aquatic animal health emergencies in Australia in an effective and efficient manner, so as to meet international and domestic policy and legal obligations concerning management of such emergencies, and coordinate national approaches to problems of public health or trade significance in animals as required."*

Not every EAD event necessitates the involvement of the CCEAD. As mentioned earlier, states and territories have sovereign powers in animal disease control within their borders. Only in certain cases would a national response be mounted, commencing with the activation of the CCEAD. Typically, the CVO (or the director of the fisheries department) of the "combat" state or territory would ask the chair of the CCEAD (the Australian CVO) to convene the CCEAD if an emergency animal disease (EAD) is suspected to be caused by a disease exotic to Australia, or if the EAD threatens to cross jurisdictional boundaries. The latter is a likely scenario for many aquatic animal diseases.

AQUAVETPLAN

The operations of the CCEAD are underpinned by *AQUAVETPLAN* – a series of response plans ("contingency plans") that describe Australia's proposed approach to an aquatic EAD event. These response plans are accompanied by technical and operational manuals and diagnostic and other training resources (Figure 1).

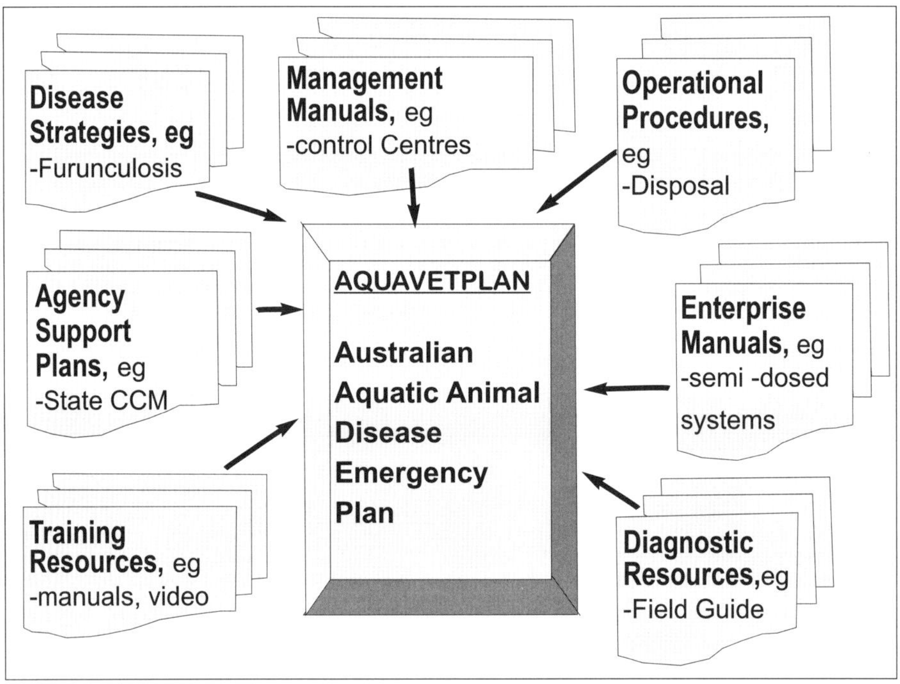

Fig. 1: The components of AQUAVETPLAN, the Australian aquatic animal disease emergency plan

To date, the following *AQUAVETPLAN* components, briefly discussed below, are freely available: operational procedure manuals, enterprise manuals, management manuals, and disease strategies.

Operational procedure manuals addressing destruction and disposal

Preventing the spread of disease might require the efficient and humane killing of stock. The manuals provide guiding principles on the decision to destroy stock and the choice and application of appropriate techniques. The safe transport and disposal of carcases, animal products, materials and wastes is also an important part of any aquatic EAD response. The manuals detail best Australian practice and provide guidance on the selection of disposal sites and methods for transportation of materials for disposal.

Enterprise manuals

The manuals guide the rapid development of aquatic EAD control strategies according to the four types of production systems affected: open (e.g. catchment, estuarine and marine); semi-open (e.g. cage cultures and shellfish); semi-closed (e.g. introduced and native freshwater fish, hatcheries and raceways); and closed (e.g. aquaria). They also provide brief information on industry practices and structures and outline approaches to be considered in the face of an aquatic EAD event.

Management manuals

Control centre management and the organisational response during the investigational, alert, operational and stand-down phases of an aquatic EAD event are outlined in the manuals and legislative, management and resource issues are addressed. The manuals list the immediate duties of field officers, senior managers, the CVO (or director of the fisheries department, where appropriate) and other staff, in each phase.

Disease strategies

Just like the terrestrial *AUSVETPLAN* disease strategy manuals, these *AQUAVETPLAN* equivalents have three sections: 1. Nature of the disease; 2. Principles of control and eradication; and 3. Preferred control policies in Australia. Figure 2 shows a typical table of contents, taken from the *AQUAVETPLAN* disease strategy for withering syndrome of abalone [7].

Currently, disease strategies are available for fish diseases (furunculosis, viral encephalopathy and retinopathy, viral haemorrhagic septicaemia, and whirling disease), mollusc diseases (withering syndrome of abalone), and crustacean diseases (crayfish plague and white spot disease).

Contents

Fig.2: Table of contents from the AQUAVETPLAN disease strategy for infection with *Candidatus* Xenohaliotis californiensis (Withering syndrome of abalone)

The *AQUAVETPLAN* series also includes agency support plans (police and local government, for example); training resources such as books and videos; and diagnostic resources. The *Aquatic Animal Diseases Significant to Australia: Identification Field Guide* was first published in 1999, with the aim of building public awareness of aquatic animal disease management in Australia. The second, revised edition was published on CD ROM in 2004 [8]. The field guide provides fisheries and aquaculture managers, aquatic veterinarians, recreational fishers, border protection staff, environmentalists and students of aquatic animal health with a quick reference guide. The field guide draws heavily on pictorial images, aiding in the rapid identification of gross signs of disease. The guide features a differential diagnostic key, directing the reader to other possible diseases as depicted by the gross signs observed. Disease reporting contacts within each Australian state and territory, as well as diagnostic links for the benefit of fish pathologists and veterinarians, are provided. The field guide was produced in consultation with members of industry, research institutes and the Australian and state and territory governments. Like all *AQUAVETPLAN* resources, this publication is available on the DAFF website (www.daff.gov.au/aquaticanimalhealth).

All *AQUAVETPLAN* manuals are developed and agreed upon in "peace time" by the Australian government, state and territory governments and relevant aquatic animal industries, to ensure that a prompt, efficient and effective response can be implemented with minimal delay. The pathway for identifying the need for a new or updated *AQUAVETPLAN* component is through a coordinated prioritisation process. At times, a need for a specific component arises and is addressed *ad hoc*. Drafts are subject to an extensive consultation and review process, and final versions are formally endorsed by governments and relevant industries.

Disease simulation exercises

AQUAVETPLAN manuals are a critical resource for a quick and effective response to aquatic EAD events. However, their usefulness relies on the extent to which involved personnel are familiar with the response plans. Also, contingency plans cannot fully cover every aspect of a real-life emergency. Therefore, practice in handling disease emergencies, including the use of existing manuals, provides the best training.

Experience in managing an emergency response can be gained in three ways: "hands-on" experience in real-life emergencies; learning from formal debriefing of real-life events; and training *via* incident simulation. All these approaches are used to increase the level of skills (including in the fields of communication, organisation, decision making, and operation) necessary for industry and government officials to quickly and effectively respond to aquatic EAD events. Disease simulation exercises can range from comparatively simple desk-top studies to complex (and resource-intensive) field exercises; can involve industry, government(s), or both; and can range across portfolios (e.g. fisheries, environment) and across jurisdictions.

Over the past several years, government officers and industry staff in Australia have participated in exercises simulating disease outbreaks in salmonids, prawns, redclaw, marron, edible oysters, pearl oysters and abalone. A multi-jurisdictional exercise, *Exercise Tethys* [1] was held in November, 2003, and simulated a concurrent disease outbreak of viral haemorrhagic septicaemia in three jurisdictions. Other jurisdictions were required to undertake necessary disease surveillance activities and participate in national decision making and resource allocation. Industry participated at the national and state levels. Virtual State Disease Control Headquarters were activated, and the aquatic CCEAD was convened [9, 10].

The outcomes of *Exercise Tethys*[1] were a set of broad recommendations aimed at improving pre-existing frameworks and resources to develop more robust communication systems and procedures for an aquatic EAD response. Additional recommendations targeted operating systems and procedures within individual jurisdictions. *Exercise Tethys*[1] also highlighted other concerns, including the need to address compensation and cost sharing issues within the aquaculture industry [10]. The recommendations were endorsed by Australia's Primary Industries Standing Committee, and a formal process is in place to monitor progress made with implementing the recommendations.

Lessons Learned And Challenges Ahead

In Australia, governments and industry have experienced that the development as well as implementation of aquatic animal health plans need proper resources. An *ad hoc* opportunistic approach to aquatic animal health funding will not be in the best interest of either industries or government. Forward planning at the strategic level is essential, with resource needs identified and agreement reached on "who provides what" and "who pays."

The two most significant problem areas encountered in establishing structural arrangements in Australia for managing aquatic animal disease emergencies were parochial attitudes and financial commitment from government and the private sector. In Australia, aquatic industries are geographically diverse (e.g., prawns in the north and north-east and salmon in the south) and share few common interests.

Likewise, state governments focus on their jurisdiction's issues rather than on national ones. Regarding financial commitment, where funding is competitive, aquatic animal health easily drops to the bottom of the priority list, both for government and industry. Also, on a global scale, Australian aquaculture is small and has little "spare cash." Providing a convincing cost-benefit analysis is inherently difficult because most benefits in the area of emergency preparedness and response accrue from things not happening.

Approaches that have proven to be successful include harmonisation with terrestrial arrangements and approaches and providing leadership with clearly identified competent authorities. Harmonisation with terrestrial approaches, has reduced the level of anxiety or "fear of the unknown"; enabled the adaptation of convincing, existing models; and minimised the duplication of efforts whilst maximising use of limited resources. While aquatic animal health does not fall into

1 Tethys was the Titanis goddess of underground fresh water. She married her brother Oceanus (the great fresh-water river that encircled the earth) and had over 3,000 children to him, they were the Potamoi (Rivers, springs and lakes of the world) and Okeanides (Clouds).

the portfolio of each state and territory CVO, the provision of national leadership through the Australian CVO was welcome and has proven to be successful. Within the Australian Government, the Office of the Australian CVO facilitates the development of national policies and strategies and the provision of scientific advice to minimise the potential impact of diseases on Australia's animal and aquatic animal health.

Deliberations with stakeholders are on-going regarding the development of, and agreement to, an aquatic Emergency Animal Disease Response Agreement (EADRA), consistent with arrangements in the terrestrial animal health sector. The terrestrial EADRA is a unique government and industry agreement that commits all parties to discharging their biosecurity responsibilities, responding to EAD events, and to a cost sharing mechanism for EAD events [see http://www.animalhealthaustralia.com.au/aahc/programs/eadp/eadra.cfm].

A similar agreement for aquatic EAD events could bring together the Australian government, state and territory governments, and aquatic industry groups. One of its possible components could be a commitment to sharing the eligible costs of the response to an aquatic EAD event. However, there is also the continuing challenge of securing an on-going funding supply to adequately support aquatic animal health management in general.

References

1. Nairn ME, Allen PG, Inglis AR, Tanner C: Australian Quarantine: a shared responsibility. Department of Primary Industries and Energy, Canberra, 1996, 284 pp.
2. Higgins RA (chair): Report of the National Task Force on Imported Fish and Fish Products. Department of Primary Industries and Energy, Canberra, Australia, 1996, 269 pp.
3. Anderson J: Australian Quarantine: a shared responsibility – The Government response. Department of Primary Industries and Energy, Canberra, Australia, 1997, 67 pp.
4. Commonwealth of Australia: AQUAPLAN – Australia's National Strategic Plan for Aquatic Animal Health 1998–2003. Australian Government Department of Agriculture, Fisheries and Forestry, Canberra, Australia, 1999, 34pp. (Accessed 22 December 2006 from http://www.daff.gov.au/aquaticanimalhealth)
5. Commonwealth of Australia: AQUAPLAN – Australia's National Strategic Plan for Aquatic Animal Health 2005-2010. Australian Government Department of Agriculture, Fisheries and Forestry. Canberra, Australia, 2005, 52 pp. (Accessed 22 December 2006 from http://www.daff.gov.au/aquaticanimalhealth).
6. Commonwealth of Australia: AQUAPLAN – A Five Year Review. Australian Government Department of Agriculture, Fisheries and Forestry, Canberra, Australia, 2002, 40pp. (Accessed 22 December 2006 from http://www.daff.gov.au/aquaticanimalhealth).
7. Department of Agriculture, Fisheries and Forestry: Disease strategy – Infection with Candidatus Xenohaliotis californiensis (withering syndrome of abalone) (Version 1.0). In Australian Government Department of Agriculture, Fisheries and Forestry: Australian Aquatic Veterinary Emergency Plan (AQUAVETPLAN). Canberra, ACT, 2006, Edition 1.0., 49 pp. (Accessed 22 December 2006 from http://www.affa.gov.au/aquaticanimalhealth).
8. Herfort A: *Aquatic Animal Diseases Significant to Australia: Identification Field Guide*. Australian Government Department of Agriculture, Fisheries and Forestry. Canberra, Australia, 2004. Accessed 22 December 2006 from http://www.disease-watch.com/documents/CD/index/index.htm).

9. East IJ, Scott KJ: Aquatic Animal Health Subprogram: design and organisation of a multi-state disease emergency simulation exercise. Fisheries Research and Development Corporation Project 2002/655. Canberra, Australia, 2004, 17 pp.
10. East IJ, Scott KJ: Aquatic Animal Health Subprogram: conduct of a multi-jurisdiction simulation exercise focused on health management in Australian aquaculture. Fisheries Research and Development Corporation Project 2003/669. Canberra, Australia, 2004, 75 pp.

Dr. Eva-Maria Bernoth, DMV, Office of the Chief Veterinary Officer, Australian Government Department of Agriculture, Fisheries and Forestry, GPO Box 858, Canberra ACT 2601, Australia.
E-mail: Eva-Maria.Bernoth@daff.gov.au

Dodet B, the OIE Scientific & Technical Department (eds): The OIE Global Conference on Aquatic Animal Health. Dev Biol (Basel). Basel, Karger, 2007, vol 129, pp 65-69.

A New System for Monitoring Health Status in Norwegian Aquaculture

K. Thorud[1], E. Brun[2], A. Lillehaug[2], M. Almklov[1], S. Romstad[3], M. Binde[3]

1 Ministry of Fisheries and Coastal Affairs, Oslo, Norway

2 National Veterinary Institute, Oslo, Norway

3 Norwegian Food Safety Authority, Oslo, Norway

Key words: aquaculture, fish health, monitoring system, Norway

Abstract: In Norway there is an official system (ANISTAT) for reporting notifiable diseases to the Norwegian Food Safety Authority, which is mainly done by veterinarians and laboratories. Another separate official system (HAVBRUKSDATA) is also in place, for reporting production data from fish farms, such as the number of fish put into the sea, and their weight, density, feed consumption and mortality. The reported data are aggregated monthly with information from companies' private databases related to each production site and each production unit. There also are official procedures in place for the registration of drugs used in aquaculture, based on veterinary prescriptions. However there is no electronic system for active reporting diseases influencing production and/or welfare.

It is our aim to establish a more advanced official system for monitoring the health situation in Norwegian fish farms (MFISK) by linking relevant production data from the various private databases to an official disease database. The output of the new system will be improved statistics on diseases in the Norwegian fish farming industry, with diseases sorted by their impact on production and welfare. This will enable us to identify diseases that, over time, cause such losses that they should be dealt with by the authorities, or by the farmers themselves. It will also have an early warning function regarding new/emerging diseases or disease trends. This system quantifies losses due to health problems and, in the long run, will be a useful tool for strengthening fish health.

The system aims to combine data from various sources: the veterinary and fisheries authorities in Norway, farmers, veterinarians and laboratories. To be sustainable, it will need the active and constructive cooperation of all these stakeholders.

INTRODUCTION

To succeed in aquaculture production it is important to have reliable knowledge and control of aquatic animal health status. A system for reporting notifiable diseases is in place and functioning in most countries, but the reporting of important diseases that are not regarded as notifiable is less obvious. In Ireland, a computerised information system was launched in the mid-1990s [1] in order to quantify the effect of various diseases and their potential risk factors. In the UK, a live fish movements database was launched in 2005 [2] in order to trace the infectious source in the case of a disease outbreak. In Norway, a summary of diagnoses from the National Veterinary Institute has been released annually for the past few years as an official report on the health situation in farmed fish [3]. Although the Veterinary Institute has a very high "market share" regarding diagnostic work in Norway, this annual report has obvious weaknesses as it is based on passive submission.

To improve our information and understanding of how fish health and welfare problems affect the industry, the idea of a new database was put forward. Three main interests were determined: to address the negative impact that fish diseases and poor fish health have on financial results for the farmers; to address the interaction between fish health and fish welfare; and to address the demand for safe products produced under ethical and sustainable production demands. This has both national and international implications and is necessary for the development and growth of the industry within the producing countries. Likewise, consumer confidence in the product is a necessary condition for gaining access and acceptance in a global market. The OIE has an important role in ensuring international standards, solidarity and transparency within this area.

HEALTH CONTROL THROUGHOUT THE PRODUCTION CHAIN

Norwegian legislation emphasizes good and continuous health control throughout the production chain: from stripping of the broodstock egg stages to the harvested fish at slaughterhouses. This control is based on three pillars. First of all, the primary basis for official health control consists of appropriate biosecurity measures throughout all stages of the production. Second, there are various sorts of surveillance conducted or imposed by the authorities. The Norwegian Food Safety Authority (NFSA) is the competent authority on animal health and welfare in Norway. It runs surveillance programmes that are aimed either at eradicating specific diseases, or declaring freedom from diseases. Just as important, is the obligation for all farmers to have routine health inspections of their farms six or 12 times a year, depending on the type and size of their production. The inspections must be conducted by veterinarians or authorized fish health biologists. They are usually organized by private, local fish health services. In addition to the routine inspections, the farms are also inspected by the fish health services in cases of increased mortality or outbreaks of disease.

When there is reason to suspect diseases that may have serious consequences, there is an obligation for everyone to report to the NFSA. Farmers and veterinarians have a particular obligation not only to report, but also to act in order to limit the consequences. The NFSA then has the power, through regulations and contingency plans, to impose further measures to limit or eradicate notifiable infectious diseases.

An Official Reporting System Containing Health Data

In Norway there are three official databases that collect health related data from aquaculture production. ANISTAT is the NFSA's database for the registration of suspected and verified notifiable diseases in fish and shellfish farms in Norway. The information in this database is the basis for official measures imposed by the NFSA in such cases. It is also the basis for international reports on notifiable diseases to the EU by the ADNS system, and to the OIE. HAVBRUKSDATA, or "AQUACULTURE DATA" is a common database for the Fisheries Authorities, Veterinary Authorities, and for the producers. HAVBRUKSDATA is a system for reporting production data from the fish farms, such as the number of fish put into sea, and their weight, density, feed consumption and mortality. The reported data are aggregated monthly with information from companies' private databases related to each production site and each production unit. There also are official procedures in place for the registration of drugs being used in aquaculture, based on veterinary prescriptions. A more advanced database for all veterinary drug prescriptions (VETREG) is under development. It is a disadvantage that there is no interoperability between the official information systems, and it is a disadvantage that there is no system for the reporting of diseases that are not notifiable.

The MFISK Monitoring System

It is our aim to establish an advanced official system for monitoring the health status of aquatic animals in Norwegian fish farms, based on private or official preexisting reporting systems and databases. A similar approach for retrieving health information has been initiated in British Columbia, Canada (Karreman G., personal communication). MFISK will be designed to give detailed and systematic documentation on the health status of fish. This implies the possibility for descriptive and exploratory statistics on diseases in Norwegian fish farming such as prevalence, incidence and spatio-temporal distribution. Combined information from all these data sources will make it possible to identify diseases that over time reduce fish health to an extent that would trigger measures from the authorities or the industry, or initiate research. This includes a possibility for the early detection of emerging diseases.

Data Input Into MFISK

When designing such a system there is a need to emphasize crucial variables that represent the main health related economic losses in Norwegian fish farming. Mortality is considered to be the most important health related loss factor. Other variables are growth rate and growth diversification and the condition and downgrading of fish at slaughter houses. Drug prescription related to outbreaks of disease or prevention of disease is considered to be a cost variable as well.

There is also a need to define variables that may explain losses, mainly disease diagnosis, different management factors and accidents (including predators). To ensure the reliability of a diagnosis its origin must be stated, whether it is a field or laboratory diagnosis. Further, there is a need to standardize most variables that enter the system.

Common diagnostic criteria need to be developed, as well as common standards for identification of the fish groups of interest for reporting. These standards should preferably be in agreement with standards that are in use in the industry. The entry and flow of the various data input in the system is depicted in Figure 1.

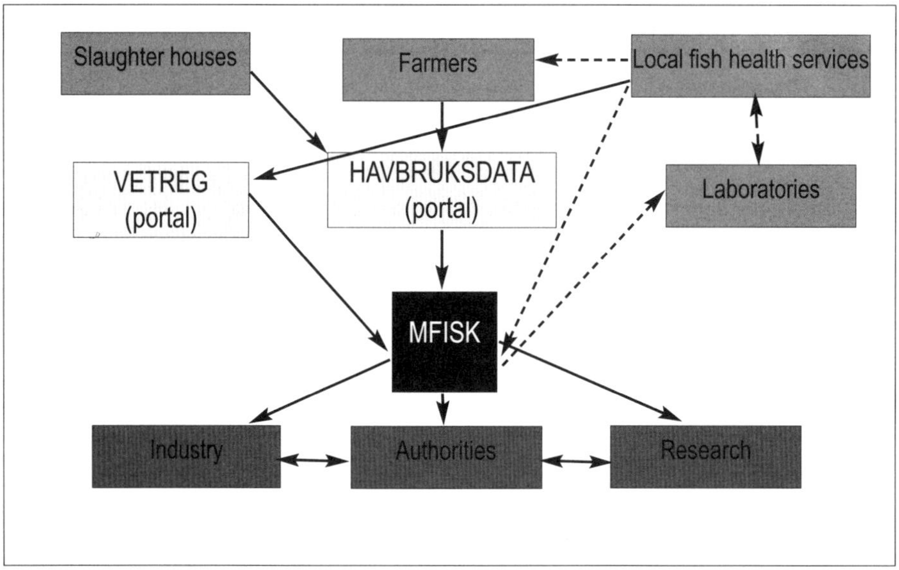

Fig.1: Data entry and flow in the MFISK system

Even if the main aim of the system is the official monitoring of fish health status, it is very important that the system is able to provide valuable information to support the industry and research. These groups should also be given restricted access to the system.

Criteria For Success

MFISK will depend upon data input from various sources. Hence it will need the cooperation of all these stakeholders. In Norway, the framework allows for requiring data that comprise the necessary input to the system. However, experience from similar work with other species in Norway tells us that it is of utmost importance that the monitoring system also is useful to those who provide the data (Larssen R.B., personal communication). That is why it is important to give the stakeholders access to valuable information from the system. The system must also be easy to use. It is crucial that it works well technically, and that it will not be too laborious to register and report reliable data. This is acknowledged by the inclusion of pre-existing industry registration documents and reports, and cooperation with stake-holders and private benchmarking systems. Finally, for MFISK to develop into a successful fish health monitoring system, it must be an interactive system where users, such as stakeholders and researchers, will apply and further improve the system.

Conclusions

The MFISK monitoring system will not only be a tool for the documentation of fish health status. It will quantify losses due to health problems and, in the long run, be a vital tool for improving fish health and welfare. It also will have an early warning function with respect to emerging and re-emerging diseases. Finally, concerning the objective of this conference, the system will have clearly defined roles and responsibilities for all stakeholders, such as the Veterinary and Fisheries Authorities, farmers, field health workers and laboratories.

References

1 Menzies FD, McLoughlin MF, Wheatley SB, Goodall EA: Development of a computerized information retrieval system for Atlantic salmon, *Salmo salar L.*, production. Aqua Res 1996; 27:183-90.

2 Hudson E, Thrush M, Oditmann B, Peeler E: Preventing and controlling notifiable exotic fish disease outbreaks in England and Wales – The role of data collection, management and analysis. EAFP 12th Int. Conf. 11-16 Sept 2005, Copenhagen.

3 Hjeltnes B (ed): The health situation in farmed fish in Norway 2006. The National Veterinary Institute, Oslo, Norway. 2007, 19 pp.

Dr. Kristin Thorud, Ministry of Fisheries and Coastal Affairs
E-mail: Kristin.Thorud@fkd.dep.no

Dodet B, the OIE Scientific & Technical Department (eds): The OIE Global Conference on Aquatic Animal Health. Dev Biol (Basel). Basel, Karger, 2007, vol 129, p 71.

Session IV

Communicating and Networking

Chairperson: *B. Hill*, UK

Dodet B, the OIE Scientific & Technical Department (eds): The OIE Global Conference on Aquatic Animal Health. Dev Biol (Basel). Basel, Karger, 2007, vol 129, pp 73-79.

Communication and Networking in a Regional Organisation

C.V. Mohan, M.J. Phillips, F. Corsin

Network of Aquaculture Centres in Asia-Pacific (NACA), Bangkok, Thailand

Key words: Network of Aquaculture Centres in Asia-Pacific (NACA), aquatic animal health, Asia Regional Technical Guidelines, intergovernmental organisation

Abstract: Access to accurate information and technical expertise is a pre-requisite for informed decision making. The Network of Aquaculture Centres in Asia-Pacific (NACA), an intergovernmental organization of 17 governments in Asia-Pacific, works on the principle of cooperation and collaboration with the intention of sharing regional resources amongst the stakeholders within the network: governments, institutions and individuals. Networking, communication and project implementation coordinated by NACA in collaboration with partner organizations and donor agencies has been instrumental in facilitating the flow of science and provision of technical assistance to relevant stakeholders in Member Countries. Development and adoption of the FAO/NACA's Asia regional technical guidelines (TG) for the responsible movement of live aquatic animals by 21 Asia-Pacific governments is a major outcome of networking and communication that had been facilitated by the NACA, from 1999 to 2001. Since then, the implementation of key elements of the TG has remained the focus of NACA's regional aquatic animal health programme. The present paper provides some examples of past and ongoing activities that highlight the role of networking and communication in a regional organization in strengthening aquatic animal health capacity and biosecurity in the Asia-Pacific region.

INTRODUCTION

The Network of Aquaculture Centres in Asia-Pacific (NACA) is an intergovernmental organization, with a current membership of 17 governments of the Asia-Pacific region, established in 1989. According to the Agreement that established the Organization, the objectives of NACA are to assist the Members in their efforts to expand aquaculture development mainly for the purpose of increasing production; improving rural income and employment; diversifying farm production; and increasing foreign exchange earnings and savings. Through six major work programmes, the NACA provides support for research cooperation, capacity building and improved communications among countries within and outside the region. Its current work programme emphasizes aquaculture for rural development, environmental sustainability and improved aquatic resources management, and is focused on poverty alleviation and food security.

The NACA operates under the principle of Technical Cooperation among Developing Countries (TCDC). The NACA program is formulated by the governments through its Governing Council, with the advice of a Technical Advisory Committee, and a wide range of government, industry and non-government stakeholders, and implemented by the Secretariat. NACA programs and projects are developed through broad participation by the stakeholders, and are (i) implemented in a participatory manner, ii) aimed at strengthening national capacities while utilizing existing regional and national institutions, (iii) designed to build on rather than duplicate results, and (iv) are shared widely

The Aquatic Animal Health Programme of the NACA

Addressing aquatic animal health is one of the key programme areas of the NACA with the purpose of assisting member governments to *"reduce the risks of aquatic animal diseases impacting the livelihoods of aquaculture farmers, national economies, trade, the environment, and human health"*. Expected outputs of the programme include improved regional and international cooperation in aquatic animal health; the development and implementation of practical national aquatic animal health strategies; improved surveillance, reporting and response to disease emergencies in the region; harmonized diagnostic procedures and approaches to risk assessment in the region; and the widespread adoption of better aquatic animal health management practices in the region.

Through the implementation of the third five-year work programme (2001-2005), considerable progress has been made in the region. Considering that different countries have achieved different levels of progress, the regional aquatic animal health program of the NACA will be further strengthened by the fourth five-year work programme (2006-2010) by focusing on the implementation of practical aquatic animal health management strategies at farm, local, national and regional levels. The sharing of experiences and resources through regional and sub-regional cooperation is being promoted through working together on common problems and improved communication, leading to more effective networking. Country specific activities built around existing resources and facilities are being initiated to develop and implement simple and practical aquatic animal heath management practices. New issues such as food safety, emerging diseases and continued introductions of exotics to the region, are being given special attention.

The following section provides some specific examples of past and ongoing activities that highlight the role of networking and communication facilitated by the NACA to further the implementation of aquatic animal health management in the Asia-Pacific region.

ASIA REGIONAL TECHNICAL GUIDELINES

With the Food and Agriculturc Organization of the United Nations (FAO), the World Organization for Animal Health (Office International des Epizooties, OIE), and with regional and international expertise, guiding principles for the responsible movement of aquatic animals and aquatic animal health management have been established. The program was initiated through an FAO regional Technical Cooperation Program project entitled "Assistance for the Responsible Movement of Live Aquatic Animals". The project was implemented between 1998 and 2001 in 21 countries and a major outcome was the *"Asia Regional Technical Guidelines on Health Management for the Responsible Movement of Live Aquatic Animals and the Beijing Consensus and Implementation Strategy"* or Technical Guidelines (TG). The guiding principles in the TG were adopted by 21 governments in the Asian region in 2000 [1]. These guidelines contain guiding principles for health management and the responsible movement of live aquatic animals that minimizes the risks of trans-boundary pathogens and diseases being introduced and spread within the Asian region. Two companion documents further support the implementation of the TG: *The Manual of Procedures* [2] and *The Asia Diagnostic Guide to Aquatic Animal Diseases* [3]. Implementation of the various components identified in the TG has been the main focus of NACA's Regional Aquatic Animal Health Program [4]. The framework provided by the TG is rather comprehensive and includes all major requirements for managing the risks associated with the movement of live aquatic animals and trans-boundary pathogens. A network of 21 National Coordinators has been guiding the process of development and implementation of national aquatic animal health strategies.

ASIA REGIONAL ADVISORY GROUP ON AQUATIC ANIMAL HEALTH

Another key element providing networking capacity within the NACA is the 10 member Regional Advisory Group (AG), which was constituted by the Governing Council of the NACA in 2001 in cooperation with the OIE and FAO with the objective of providing advice to NACA and Asian governments on aquatic animal health management. The AG meets on an annual basis to review the Asian disease situation, consider regional and international developments and develop and communicate specialist advice to governments on aquatic animal health management matters. The fifth meeting of the AG [5] was held in November, 2006. The NACA facilitates the implementation of the mandate of the AG and works closely with the OIE and FAO to promote the role of the region in influencing international standard setting and trade policies. The report from the AG, for example, is now considered at the OIE Aquatic Animal Health Standards Commission, providing specialist information from the region to this global OIE standard setting body.

Quarterly Aquatic Animal Disease (QAAD) Reporting System

The QAAD reporting system in the Asia-Pacific region has been implemented as a joint activity between the NACA, FAO and OIE Regional Representation (Tokyo) since the second quarter of 1998. To date, 34 QAAD reports have been published and widely disseminated [6]. Twenty-one countries from the region participate in the reporting system. The QAAD list includes all diseases listed by OIE in the latest edition of the OIE *Aquatic Animal Health Code*, plus diseases of concern to the Asia-Pacific region. The regional QAAD reporting system provides up-to-date information on important diseases in the Asia-Pacific region, serves as an early warning system for emerging diseases and is a valuable source of information to support risk analysis. To ensure effective implementation at the national level, governments have designated National Coordinators (NC) for each of the participating governments. The NCs organise the surveillance and disease reporting systems for reportable diseases and prepare QAAD reports. Since 2001, the QAAD list has been revised annually by the AG. The revisions are carried out to reflect the changes made to the OIE list of aquatic animal diseases as shown in the latest edition of the OIE *Aquatic Animal Health Code*, and to include diseases of concern to the Asia-Pacific region. As a result of these revisions, the regional QAAD list has contributed to listing of some serious emerging diseases (e.g., infection with koi herpes virus, abalone viral mortality, grouper iridoviral disease, white tail disease in *Macrobrachium rosenbergii*, and infectious myonecrosis virus).

Regional Resource Base

One way to support the implementation of responsible health management is to effectively use the vast pool of technical expertise that is available in the region. In this direction, NACA has embarked on a new regional initiative – *identifying and establishing a three tier regional resource base* - to utilize the technical resources available in the region for the benefit of its member countries. The first resource level is made of Regional Resource Experts (RRE) who contribute their expertise through answering technical questions related to their field of expertise; assisting in development of disease cards, diagnostic manuals and supporting documents; and providing diagnostic assistance as far as possible during disease emergencies. The second resource level, the Regional Resource Centres (RRC), supports the initiative through the provision of scientific and technical training for personnel from the region; the provision of diagnostic testing facilities to countries who are members of the regional aquatic animal health initiative and their personnel; and the organisation of scientific meetings, training courses and re-training workshops on behalf of the NACA. The third resource level, the Regional Reference Laboratories (RRL) for diseases of regional concern not listed by the OIE, provides centres of expertise and standardization for designated diseases. Good progress has already been made and the current list of RREs, RRCs and RRLs within this initiative can be found at www.enaca.org. The regional resource base is increasingly used by stakeholders in Member Countries.

Risk Analysis

Recognizing the importance of scientific risk analysis in minimizing the risk of the introduction and spread of trans-boundary pathogens/diseases, an APEC Fisheries Working Group-funded project, APEC FWG 01/2002, "Capacity and Awareness Building on IRA for Aquatic Animals," was successfully implemented by the NACA from 2002 to 2004 in partnership with several regional and international organizations. Two training workshops brought together regulatory authorities and administrators responsible for the trade of live aquatic animals, and aquatic animal health specialists, to share experiences, raise awareness, build capacity, and contribute to the development of a practical manual for risk analysis to support responsible aquatic animal movements [7,8].

Sub-Regional Networking

AusAid, under the Association of Southeast Asian Nations (ASEAN)-Australia Development Cooperation Program's Regional Partnership Scheme (AADCP-RPS) is currently supporting two aquatic animal health projects: Strengthening Aquatic Animal Health Capacity and Biosecurity in ASEAN and Operationalise Guidelines on Responsible Movement of Live Food Finfish in ASEAN. These projects have been in operation since January, 2006, and directly support capacity building, harmonization and the facilitation of trade within the ASEAN. The goal of the first project is to enhance the capability of ASEAN Member Countries to implement ASEAN harmonized national aquatic animal health strategies to manage risks to the biosecurity of fisheries industries, particularly those related to trade and impacting on the poor. The project will support the development of harmonized approaches to aquatic animal health management and biosecurity in ASEAN and increasing capacity to implement the ASEAN harmonized national aquatic animal health and biosecurity strategies. The second project aims to enhance the biosecurity of food finfish industries in ASEAN Member Countries by reducing the risk of the international spread of specific fish pathogens and developing harmonized standard operating procedures for health certification and quarantine measures for the transboundary movement of live food finfish within ASEAN. Project activities (e.g., four workshops, two training programs and four technical missions) involving over 60 delegates from 10 ASEAN countries would result in the establishement of a strong regional network amongst ASEAN countries and contribute to improved communication.

Recently, the NACA has initiated consultations with the South Asia Association for Regional Cooperation (SAARC) to discuss opportunities for cooperation on aquatic animal health in this important sub-region.

Other Project Activities

In addition to the above examples, specific project driven networking activities facilitated and/or coordinated by the NACA have immensely contributed to the strengthening of the regional health program through capacity building (e.g., diagnostics, epidemiology, sampling, surveillance, risk analysis, and contingency planning); the development of resource material (e.g., technical guidelines, manuals, diagnostic guides, field identification guides, disease cards, extension brochures, etc.); the provision of technical assistance to individual countries (e.g., technical missions to assist in the development of national strategies); the development of standard operating procedures (e.g. SOPs, for the responsible movement of live food finfish within ASEAN); the harmonization of methods (e.g., PCR inter-calibration exercise in India and Indonesia); the development of diagnostics (e.g., ACIAR supported shrimp regional project); and promoting the adoption of better aquatic animal health management practices (e.g. shrimp better management practice (BMP) projects in India, Vietnam, Thailand and Indonesia).

Conclusions

Networking established in the Asia-Pacific region under the NACA umbrella has been successful in building awareness and capacity at different levels, including farmers, by facilitating the flow of science and providing appropriate technical assistance for informed decision making. Networking facilitates a free flow of knowledge and ideas which can sometimes be more important than the transfer of packaged information and which also very cheaply facilitates the development of information products and their subsequent updates. NACA networking has included institutions and experts from all over the world, facilitating the flow of knowledge, technology and ideas between regional researchers and colleagues from other regions, with uncountable positive implications.

References

1 FAO/NACA (Food and Agriculture Organization of the United Nations/Network of Aquaculture Centres in Asia-Pacific): Asia Regional Technical Guidelines on Health Management for the Responsible Movement of Live Aquatic Animals and the Beijing Consensus and Implementation Strategy: FAO Fisheries Technical Paper No. 402. FAO, Rome, 2000.

2 FAO/NACA (Food and Agriculture Organization of the United Nations/Network of Aquaculture Centres in Asia-Pacific): Manual of Procedures for the Implementation of the Asia Regional Technical Guidelines on Health Management for the Responsible Movement of Live Aquatic Animals. FAO Fisheries Technical Paper No. 402, Suppl. 1. FAO, Rome, 2001.

3 Bondad-Reantaso, M.G., S.E. McGladdery, I. East, R.P. Subasinghe, (eds): Asia Diagnostic Guide to Aquatic Animal Diseases. FAO Fisheries Technical Paper, No. 402, Suppl. 2. FAO, Rome, 2001.

4 Mohan CV, Bondad-Reantaso MG: Regional approach to aquatic animal health management-views and programmes of Network of Aquaculture Centres in Asia-Pacific, in In D.Scarfe, Lee, C.S, O'Bryen, P (eds). Aquaculture Biosecurity: Prevention, control and eradication of aquatic animal disease. Blackwell Publishing, 2006, pp 17-29.

5 NACA (Network of Aquaculture Centres in Asia-Pacific): Report of the Fifth Meeting of the Asia Regional Advisory Group on Aquatic Animal Health: NACA, Bangkok, 2007.

6 NACA/FAO (Network of Aquaculture Centres in Asia-Pacific/Food and Agriculture Organization of the United Nations): Quarterly Aquatic Animal Disease Report (Asia and Pacific Region), July-September 2006. NACA, Bangkok, 2007 http://www.enaca.org/modules/wfsection/article.php?articleid=7).

7 Arthur JR, Bondad-Reantaso MG, Baldock FC, Rodgers CJ, Edgerton BF: Manual on Risk Analysis for the Safe Movement of Aquatic Animals (FWG/01/2002): APEC/DoF/NACA/FAO, NACA, Bangkok, 2004.

8 Arthur JR, Bondad-Reantaso MG (eds): Capacity and Awareness Building on Import Risk Analysis (IRA) for Aquatic Animals: Proceedings of the Workshops, 1-6 April 2002, Bangkok, Thailand and 12-17 August 2002, Mazatlan, Mexico. Asia-Pacific Economic Cooperation Fisheries Working Group (APEC FWG) 01/2002, NACA, Bangkok, 2004.

Dr. C.V. Mohan, Network of Aquaculture Centres in Asia-Pacific (NACA), Suraswadi Building, Department of Fisheries, Kasetsart University Campus, Ladyao, Jatujak, Bangkok 10900, Thailand.
E-mail: mohan@enaca.org

Dodet B, the OIE Scientific & Technical Department (eds): The OIE Global Conference on Aquatic Animal Health. Dev Biol (Basel). Basel, Karger, 2007, vol 129, pp 81-89.

International Disease Reporting and Communication

D. Chaisemartin

Head of the Administrative and Management System Department, World Organisation for Animal Health (OIE), Paris, France.

Key words: disease, aquatic animal, disease reporting, disease communication, world animal health information system

Abstract: The transparency of the world aquatic animal health situation is based on formal information provided to the OIE through notification by Member Countries when a disease event occurs within their territory. The efficiency of this transparency has been increased since 2002 by the addition of the active search and verification of unofficial information based on various sources. This system is also completed by the exchange of unofficial information between FAO, the OIE and WHO in the context of the GLEWS agreement. Other improvements consist of the establishment, in 2004, of new criteria for listing OIE diseases on a single list, and modification of the notification procedures, in 2005. The OIE World Animal Health Information System has been modernised with the web application WAHIS. The communication of information has also been improved thanks to an electronic distribution list that has been created for Delegates, OIE partners, the general public or institutions interested in receiving alert messages and weekly newsletters. The use of mapping to describe disease distribution worldwide has also been introduced on the website. The website has also been modernised with the development of the WAHID Interface, the new interface of the World Animal Health Information System Database, which allows end-users to perform a wide range of queries for a given country and a given disease. The international aquatic animal disease database of the CEFAS (OIE Collaborating Centre) allows the public to access official information from the OIE and other information found in publications.

INTRODUCTION

One of the historical missions of the OIE is to ensure transparency in the world animal disease situation including regarding zoonoses. Member Countries have to report animal diseases detected on their territory to the OIE. When the OIE receives new information from a Member Country, it distributes it for necessary preventive action. The diffusion of information regarding the animal disease situation is done through the OIE website, by e-mail for the alert messages and weekly disease information bulletins, and via publications.

THE OIE GLOBAL ANIMAL HEALTH INFORMATION SYSTEM

The OIE Global Animal Health Information System is composed of three main elements. The first is the OIE Early Warning System, based on the official information sent by Member Countries and the report sent by the OIE Reference Laboratories. Member Countries are obliged to report diseases, emerging diseases or pathogenic agents with epidemiological significance to other countries according to the conditions described in the chapter on notification and epidemiological information (Chapter 1.2.1. of the *Aquatic Animal Health Code*) to the OIE Central Bureau. The second element is a monitoring system based on the official information sent by Member Countries concerning the animal health situation regarding OIE listed diseases or infections. This includes a six-monthly and annual report sent to the OIE as described in the chapter on notification and epidemiological information indicated above. Finally, there is the active search and verification of unofficial information sent by ProMed or GPHIN, found in scientific publications, in the news or with some tools like Copernic. When unofficial information is found, it is analysed by the animal health information department. If the information is already known, no action is required. If the information is new, the data is checked on the OIE databases. Two cases might arise. If it is a disease in a country without a new epidemiological event, no action is required. If it is a new event, based on the article 1.2.1.3. of the *Aquatic Animal Health Code*, an official letter is sent to the OIE Delegate for confirmation and additional data. The OIE regularly contacts the Delegate until a response is received. The official response is analysed. If the answer does not confirm the unofficial information, the procedure is ended. If the answer confirms the unofficial information, the country has to do an immediate notification and the follow-up reports and data are shared with other services of the OIE and the organisations (FAO, WHO) concerned within the Global Early Warning System and Response (GLEWS) framework. GLEWS is the FAO/OIE/WHO joint initiative regarding the exchange of official and unofficial data for a list of fifteen priority animal diseases including zoonoses and emerging diseases, with verification of unofficial data. Since 2002, there has been an increase in unofficial data found and letters sent out. Active research was responsible for the recognition of eighteen immediate notifications in 2002, 14 in 2003, 39 in 2004 and 36 in 2005.

History of the New World Animal Health Information System

At the General Session in May, 2003, the OIE Delegates approved the move to a single disease listing. Following the adoption of this resolution, an *ad hoc* group was created to discuss the definition of criteria for including and excluding an OIE listed disease. The results were proposed to the International Committee and, during the General Session in May, 2004, resolutions were adopted regarding the criteria for placing a disease on the OIE list (terrestrial animal), with the conception of the new animal heath information system. The International Committee agreed to merge list A and list B to form a single OIE list for 2005. New forms of notification were discussed by an *ad hoc* group in July, 2004. The technical specifications for the computing system of the new World Animal Health Information System (WAHIS) were written in 2004 and a call for tenders was made for the selection of a company to develop the WAHIS application and the web interface (WAHID interface: World Animal Health Information Database interface). This application was developed during the years 2005 and 2006 and the WAHIS internet system was launched in April, 2006, with the annual report added in August 2006.

The Obligation of Member Countries

Through the OIE, countries should make accessible all information necessary to minimise the spread of aquatic animal diseases and assist in achieving better global control of these diseases. To achieve this, countries must comply with the required reports. Veterinary Administrations must send immediate notification (within 24 hours), by fax or e-mail, of any of the following events to the OIE: the first occurrence or re-occurrence of an OIE listed disease in a country if the country was previously considered to be free of that particular disease; if an OIE listed disease has occurred in a new host species; if an OIE listed disease has occurred with a new pathogen strain or in a new disease manifestation; if an OIE listed disease has newly recognised zoonotic potential; or if there is a case of an emerging disease or pathogenic agent with findings that are of epidemiological significance to other countries.

In deciding whether findings justify immediate notification (within 24 hours), countries must ensure that they comply with the obligations of Section 1.3. of the *Aquatic Animal Health Code* (especially Article 1.3.1.1.), to report developments that may have implications for international trade.

Weekly reports must also be sent to the OIE, by fax or e-mail, subsequent to a notification described above, to provide further information on the evolution of the incident that justified immediate notification. These reports should continue until the disease has been eradicated or the situation has become sufficiently stable that six-monthly reporting as described below will satisfy the obligation of the country to the OIE; in each case, a final report on the incident should be submitted.

Six-monthly reports on the absence or presence and evolution of OIE listed diseases, and findings of epidemiological significance to other countries with respect to diseases that are not listed, must be sent to the OIE. Finally, Member Countries must send the OIE an annual report concerning any other information of significance to other countries.

The OIE Listed Diseases

Diseases proposed for the OIE list must meet all of the relevant parameters set for each of the criteria, namely A. Consequences, B. Spread and C. Diagnosis. Therefore, to be listed, a disease must have the following characteristics described in Table 1: 1 or 2 or 3; and 4 or 5; and 6-8.

Table 1a: Criteria for OIE listed diseases

No. A. Consequences	Criteria (A-C)	Parameters that support a listing	Explanatory notes
1.		The disease has been shown to cause significant production losses at a national or multinational (zone or regional) level.	There is a general pattern that the disease will lead to losses in susceptible species, and that morbidity or mortality are related primarily to the agent and not management or environmental factors. (Morbidity includes, for example, loss of production due to spawning failure.) The direct economic impact of the disease is linked to its morbidity, mortality and effect on product quality.
2.	Or	The disease has been shown to or scientific evidence indicates that it is likely to negatively affect wild aquatic animal populations that are an asset worth protecting for economic or ecological reasons.	Wild aquatic animal populations can be populations that are commercially harvested (wild fisheries) and hence are an economic asset. However, the asset could be ecological or environmental in nature, for example, if the population consists of an endangered species of aquatic animal or an aquatic animal potentially endangered by the disease.
3.	Or	The agent is of public health concern.	
4.		Infectious aetiology of the disease is proven.	

Table 1b: Criteria for OIE listed diseases

And **B. Spread**			
5.	Or	An infectious agent is strongly associated with the disease, but the aetiology is not yet known.	Infectious diseases of unknown aetiology can have equally high-risk implications as those diseases where the infectious aetiology is proven. Whilst disease occurrence data are gathered, research should be conducted to elucidate the aetiology of the disease and the results be made available within a reasonable period of time.
6.	And	Potential for international spread, including via live animals, their products or fomites.	International trade in aquatic animal species susceptible to the disease exists or is likely to develop and, under international trading practices, the entry and establishment of the disease is a likely risk.
7.	And	Several countries or countries with zones may be declared free of the disease based on the general surveillance principles outlined in Chapter 1.1.4 of the *Manual of Diagnostic Tests for Aquatic Animals.*	Free countries/zones could still be protected. Listing of diseases that are ubiquitous or extremely widespread would render notification unfeasible. However, individual countries that run a control programme on such a disease can demand its listing provided they have undertaken a scientific evaluation to support their request. Examples may be the protection of broodstock from widespread diseases, or the protection of the last remaining free zones from a widespread disease.
And **C. Diagnosis**			
8.		A repeatable, robust means of detection/diagnosis exists.	A diagnostic test should be widely available and preferably has undergone a formal standardisation and validation process using routine field samples (see Manual of Diagnostic Tests for Aquatic Animals) or a robust case definition is available to clearly identify cases and allow them to be distinguished from other pathologies.

The OIE aquatic animal listed diseases are listed in Table 2.

Table 2: OIE aquatic animal listed diseases

Diseases of fish
Epizootic haematopoietic necrosis
Infectious haematopoietic necrosis
Spring viremia of carp
Viral haemorrhagic septicaemia
Infectious salmon anaemia
Epizootic ulcerative syndrome
Gyrodactylosis (*Gyrodactylus salaris*)
Red sea bream iridoviral disease
Koi herpesvirus disease
Diseases of molluscs
Infection with *Bonamia ostreae*
Infection with *Bonamia exitiosa*
Infection with *Marteilia refringens*
Infection with *Perkinsus marinus*
Infection with *Perkinsus olseni*
Infection with *Xenohaliotis californiensis*
Abalone viral mortality
Diseases of crustaceans
Taura syndrome
White spot disease
Yellowhead disease
Tetrahedral baculovirosis (*Baculovirus penaei*)
Spherical baculovirosis (Penaeus monodon-type baculovirus)
Infectious hypodermal and haematopoietic necrosis
Crayfish plague (*Aphanomyces astaci*)
Necrotising hepatopancreatitis (Under study)
Infectious myonecrosis (Under study)

A newly recognised disease or a known disease behaving differently may be listed if it meets the following criteria (1 or 2, and 3 or 4) in Table 3.

Table 3: Criteria for listing a new disease

No.	Parameters that support a listing	Explanatory notes
1.	Infectious aetiology of the disease is proven.	
Or		
2.	An infectious agent is strongly associated with the disease, but the aetiology is not yet known.	Infectious diseases of unknown aetiology can have equally high-risk implications as those diseases where the infectious aetiology is proven. Whilst disease occurrence data are gathered, research should be conducted to elucidate the aetiology of the disease and the results be made available within a reasonable period of time.
And		
3.	The agent is of public health concern.	
Or		
4.	Significant spread in naive populations of wild or cultured aquatic animals.	The disease has exhibited significant morbidity, mortality or production losses at a zone, compartment or country level. 'Naive' means animals previously unexposed either to a new disease or a new form of a known disease.

New manuals and forms were created in order to standardize notification and specify the required data. The new World Animal Health Information System allows for registration of all the different reports that the countries have to send in order to ensure transparency with respect to the global animal disease and zoonosis situation.

The Components of the Reports

Immediate notification and follow-up reports

When a new OIE listed disease, an emerging disease or a pathogenic agent with epidemiological significance to other countries appears, the country in which it appears has to make an immediate notification which must contain the following information: the reason for the notification; the date of the report, the date in which the event started, and confirmation date of the event; the nature of the diagnosis; the details regarding the occurrences by first administrative division with the location, type of the epidemiological unit, geographical coordinates, date of the incident, the species concerned and the associated data (number of susceptible animals, number of cases, number of deaths, number of destroyed animals, and number of slaughtered animals); control measures undertaken or to be undertaken; the source of the occurrences or origin of the infection; and possible laboratory tests made to confirm the infection or disease.

After an immediate notification, every week the Delegate will send a follow-up report which updates the components of the immediate notification, in particular the occurrences, control measures undertaken or to be undertaken, the source of the occurrences or origin of the infection and the laboratory tests. The Delegate will send a final report when the event is ended or when the amplitude of the event increases to the point of becoming endemic.

Routine Reports

Every six months, the Member Countries must report on the animal health situation concerning all OIE listed diseases. The six-monthly report contains two sections. First, there is a section including qualitative information and the following elements: date of the report; disease occurrence; control, prophylaxis and prevention measures; and an indication of the type of report to be used to notify diseases or infections present in the country. If the disease is absent or no information is available, it is not necessary to indicate the type of report to be used. If a disease is present or suspected, it is necessary to indicate only one type of report to be used (choice between four templates). There is a section including quantitative information which contains the different form templates. Template 1 regards the details of the occurrences by first administrative division and by month. This template is recommended for the diseases which are notifiable within the country. Template 2 regards the details of the occurrences for the whole country by month. Template 3 regards the details of the occurrences by first administrative division for a six month period. Template 4 regards the details of the occurrences for the whole country for a six month period. Each template contains the following elements: the number of new occurrences, the total number of occurrences, the species concerned and the associated data (number of susceptible animals, number of cases, number of deaths, number of destroyed animals, and number of slaughtered animals).

After the end of the year, the Delegate has to send an OIE/FAO/WHO annual report. A new form for the annual report was created in January 2006. This report contains the following elements: OIE and non-OIE listed diseases for countries which are not members of the OIE (disease occurrence and the associated data for the whole country and the six-month period); OIE listed diseases for the OIE Member Countries; human cases and human deaths for OIE listed zoonotic diseases; veterinarians and animal health technicians; national reference laboratories; and vaccine production.

The New World Animal Health Information System

The new World Animal Health Information System allows for the registration of all the different reports the Delegates must send to the OIE. The system uses maps and geographic coordinates for describing the location of the outbreaks. Access (via login and password) will be available to each Delegate. When accessing the system for the first time, the Delegate must check the first administrative unit used by the veterinary services. Delegates can nominate a person responsible for notifying diseases or infections in terrestrial or aquatic animals. Notifications include immediate notification, the follow-up report, six-monthly report and the annual report. For better management of the reports, each nominee registered by the Delegate receives a login and password in order to access WAHIS.

For each kind of report, the new World Animal Health Information System allows the Delegate or the nominee to save a draft, print a report, save it on the computer and transmit it to the OIE. The Delegate or the nominee can edit existing reports. For the six-monthly report, the system includes data that has already been reported for a given period for the diseases which have been notified. The six-monthly and annual reports can be also made in several steps. Fifty countries have already used WAHIS to send the OIE their six-monthly report.

Dissemination of Information

After receiving data from a country, the dissemination of information is done through the OIE website, by e-mail for the alert messages and the weekly disease information bulletin, and via publications. A new Web interface, named WAHID, will be displayed in a few months. Of course, at the beginning, the OIE website will show the data on the Handistatus interface for years before 2006 and on the WAHID interface for years thereafter.

The WAHID interface will contain the following items: a summary and detailed information about a specified country, including disease event reports, animal health status, veterinary services, population, and vaccination; information about a particular disease, including global status maps, outbreak maps, and lists of countries with different statuses; lists and maps of the prophylactic and control measures used by country and by disease; and a comparison of the animal health status of two countries for trade purposes. This identifies which diseases may pose a hazard for countries importing animals or animal products from another country

The website of the OIE Collaborating Centre for information on aquatic animal diseases, the Cefas Weymouth Laboratory, displays an international database on aquatic animal diseases. The development and maintenance of this database is entirely funded by the DEFRA (Department for Environment, Food and Rural Affairs) in the United Kingdom. This database shows the occurrence of OIE listed diseases, including the official data received and published by the OIE and unofficial data found in publications. This database also shows the existing data for aquatic animal diseases which were previously on the OIE list.

Dr. Daniel Chaisemartin, Head of the Administrative and Management System Department, World Organisation for Animal Health (OIE) 12, rue de Prony 75017 Paris, France
E-mail: d.chaisemartin@oie.int

Dodet B, the OIE Scientific & Technical Department (eds): The OIE Global Conference on Aquatic Animal Health. Dev Biol (Basel). Basel, Karger, 2007, vol 129, pp 91-102.

Refinement and Use of Certificates of Veterinary Inspection (Health Certificates) for Optimal Assurance of Disease Freedom in Aquatic Animals

D.E. Starling[1], D. Palić[2], A.D. Scarfe[3]

1 Aqueterinary Services, PC, Boone, IA, USA

2 Center for Food Security and Public Health, Iowa State University, Ames, IA, USA

3 American Veterinary Medical Association, Schaumburg, IL, USA

Key words: certificate of veterinary inspection (CVI), health certificate, aquatic animal, model

Abstract: Certificates of Veterinary Inspection (CVI), generally termed “Health Certificates”, are pivotal for ensuring that translocated animals are not diseased or do not harbour significant pathogens. While used very successfully with terrestrial animal movement for decades, CVIs for aquatic animals are not well refined, understood or used, despite the availability of several aquatic animal “certification processes”, “permits” and “health certificates”, including the OIE model health certificates. Correctly designed CVIs provide the single most economical and effective assurance of disease status (generally freedom from specific diseases or pathogens) for individuals or lots of animals, at any point in time. When issued by a qualified independent third-party (typically a licensed and government accredited veterinarian) they provide the official level of assurance necessary for intrastate, interstate and international trade. Tailored modifications of CVIs are also useful for other purposes requiring the evaluation of animal health (e.g. specific pathogen-free (SPF) assurance for premises, risk-mitigating assurance necessary for insurance policies, breeding soundness assurance of broodstock, etc.). Here we discuss necessary information for aquatic animal CVIs: animal, ownership and location; standardized diagnostic results and their interpretation; and language contained in CVIs. Also addressed is the viability for use with multiple aquatic species and diseases/pathogens of interest, and their use in conjunction with established veterinary inspection procedures. A revised model aquatic CVI, with broad potential use for individual operations, states or countries, is offered for discussion, comment and refinement. In addition an optimally designed model CVI may be of use with electronic systems that are evolving in, for example, Europe, the USA and Australia/New Zealand (e.g. TRACES, e-CVI, e-Certs).

Introduction

Globally, aquaculture is steadily expanding both with regard to total production and the range of species farmed. With overall annual growth close to 10%, aquaculture is by far the fastest growing sector of food animal production in the world and is providing an increased proportion of the total production of fish and shellfish for human consumption. Aquatic animals and their products are widely traded and their international trade has continued to expand at an annual growth rate of about 4% in recent years [1]. It has been estimated that 195 countries export part of their fisheries and/or aquaculture and the net trade surplus for developing countries has increased to almost 20 billion $US, illustrating the importance of the export trade [2]. The international trade is not confined only to aquaculture animals and products for human consumption, but there is also rise in the production of farmed ornamental fish, as well as increase in the wild capture and transport of tropical varieties for the pet trade, often with damaging effects on native populations [3].

The transport of live aquatic animals (including eggs, water, and containers) has been a necessity for much of the expansion of the aquaculture and companion fish sectors, but it has also contributed significantly to the occurrence and spread of economically serious diseases in the industry. In many countries (developed and undeveloped alike), the rapid increase in aquaculture output has been based on species diversification that has led to an increase in the introduction and transfer of live, non-indigenous aquatic animals for farming [2]. Furthermore, until recently tropical fish trade has not been regarded as posing a significant disease risk to either aquaculture or wild aquatic animals, and has mostly been unrestricted by import health certification requirements in importing countries [1]. Recent changes in the regulation of the aquatic animal trade in the UK, and some other countries have addressed this issue. Tropical and temperate ornamental fish trade (koi carp and goldfish) have recently been implicated in the spread of certain diseases of farmed and wild fish, but only a few countries have applied health certification requirements on import. The spread of disease is causing significant economic losses in international aquaculture production and has a detrimental effect on export trade [1]. Despite certain efforts, diseases continue to spread internationally even where import health safeguards are in place; although local pathogens, inadequate farm management, environmental factors and poor water quality continue to be most common causes of disease outbreaks in farmed fish and shellfish, the transfer of pathogens due to international trade in live aquatic animals and their products is a major underlying reason for new disease occurrences in importing countries [2,4,5].

A Certificate of Veterinary Inspection (CVI, as utilized in terrestrial animal transport and trade) is an official document, issued and signed by a licensed veterinarian in the country or state of origin. The CVI provides documentation that an animal or a group of animals was apparently healthy and showed no signs of contagious or communicable diseases in an environment of low disease risk on the date the inspection took place [6]. CVIs (generally, but less precisely also termed "Health Certificates"), are pivotal for ensuring that translocated animals are not diseased or do not harbour significant pathogens [4,7]. Correctly designed and used CVIs provide the single most economical and effective assurance of the disease status (generally, freedom from specific diseases or pathogens) for individuals or lots of animals, at any point in time. When issued by a qualified independent third-party (typically a licensed veterinarian, and in some countries under government accreditation) they provide an official level of assurance necessary for intrastate, interstate and international trade. With modifications tailored to specific purposes, CVIs are also extremely useful for other disease-related purposes requiring evaluation of animal health including specific pathogen-free (SPF) assurance for premises, risk-mitigating (biosecurity practices) assurance necessary for insurance policies, and the assurance of broodstock breeding soundness.

While used very successfully with terrestrial animal movement for decades, CVIs for aquatic animals are not well refined, understood or used, despite the availability of several aquatic animal "certification processes", "permits", and "health certificates", including the OIE model health certificates. Necessary categories of information for aquatic animal CVIs, including animal, ownership and location, standardized diagnostic results and their interpretation, and language contained in CVIs are described, and their viability for use with multiple aquatic species and diseases/pathogens of interest is presented in conjunction with established veterinary inspection procedures. A revised model aquatic CVI, with broad potential use for individual operations, states or countries, is offered for discussion, comment and refinement. In addition, opportunities for an optimally designed model CVI to be used with electronic systems that are evolving in Europe, the USA and Australia/New Zealand (e.g. TRACES, e-CVI, e-Certs) are discussed.

Although several "health certificate" templates exist today, including the OIE model, [4] there is major distinction between health certificate and certificate of veterinary inspection (CVI). Health certificates can be produced and presented via competent authorities in the country of origin, including licensed veterinary professionals, while CVIs are exclusively done by licensed and often accredited veterinarians. In terrestrial animal transport and trade, CVIs are only issued by licensed veterinarians in any country with existing veterinary infrastructure, however, the aquatic animals transport and trade sector has not invited or utilized "conventional" veterinary medicine to the same extent. Therefore, alongside the regulatory veterinary services, different authorities can be in charge of the control and certification of aquatic animal health [4,7]. Although education efforts in aquatic veterinary medicine in the US and the European Union have partly offset the past lack of trained veterinary workforce [8], the rapid increase in production volume and globalization of aquatic animal trade and transport has only recently been followed by the larger scale introduction of aquatic animal education programs for veterinarians [9]. Nevertheless, the combination of industry expansion and emergence and the devastating impact of various known and new diseases in aquatic animals has called for and supported the increased presence of the veterinary profession in aquatic animal medicine in order to help the industry and protect international trade, using the same principles well established in terrestrial animal species. Probably the most important distinction is that while veterinary para-professionals and experts in aquatic animal diseases without veterinary medical background are an irreplaceable part of aquatic animal science, husbandry and education, no one but the licensed veterinarian can produce a certificate of veterinary inspection. The major problem that can be associated with issuance of CVIs is that some developing and in-transition countries, as well as less developed regulatory agencies, lack the infrastructure to support the services of practicing veterinarians, especially in aquatic animal medicine. Non-veterinary-service authorities (or "competent authorities") often have the regulatory purview to issue health certificates for aquatic animals. Therefore, the proposed model for the aquatic CVI has the flexibility to function as a guiding foundation and ultimate goal for the present certification systems limited to utilizing "health certificates" until the regulatory authority and industry infrastructure support a complete Certificate of Veterinary Inspection, provided that the title of the document and government endorsement will clearly distinguish the document used for this purpose.

Model Aquatic Animal Certificate of Veterinary Inspection

Necessary information captured in an aquatic animal model CVI (Fig.1) includes several major components such as the header, source and destination, animal information, required laboratory disease diagnostic tests, declarations, and endorsements. Other information specific for the conditions of the trade agreement, or the issuing institution or country can be embedded in the existing format.

It is the author's opinion that the term "Certificate of Veterinary Inspection" should be used specifically for the document issued by veterinarians or veterinary authority as a distinction of infrastructure evolution, while term "Health Certificate" can be used by non-veterinary competent authorities. In this text, the abbreviation "CVI" will be used and considered interchangeable with the term "health certificate" when issued by veterinarians or the competent veterinary authority. The following sections of the document are proposed for consideration by veterinary regulatory authorities and other competent authorities, as well as various institutions and industry associations.

Section 1, the heading section, will include identification of the veterinary authority that is issuing the CVI, with the authority's contact information and unique authority identification number for document control purposes. A CVI may be issued as a declaration of examination/testing results for an individual animal, lot/group of animals; or a statement of inspection about a facility/premises suitability to a specific function or use, or other such purposes; with the reason for issuance of the CVI stated in the "issued for" section. Due to the huge diversity of aquatic animals used for aquaculture and trade (finfish, shellfish, crustaceans, molluscs, amphibians, reptiles…), the "animal type" needs to be clearly identified on the CVI. Finally, "the statement of CVI purpose" (sale, movement, breeding, insurance, other…) concludes the header part of the CVI.

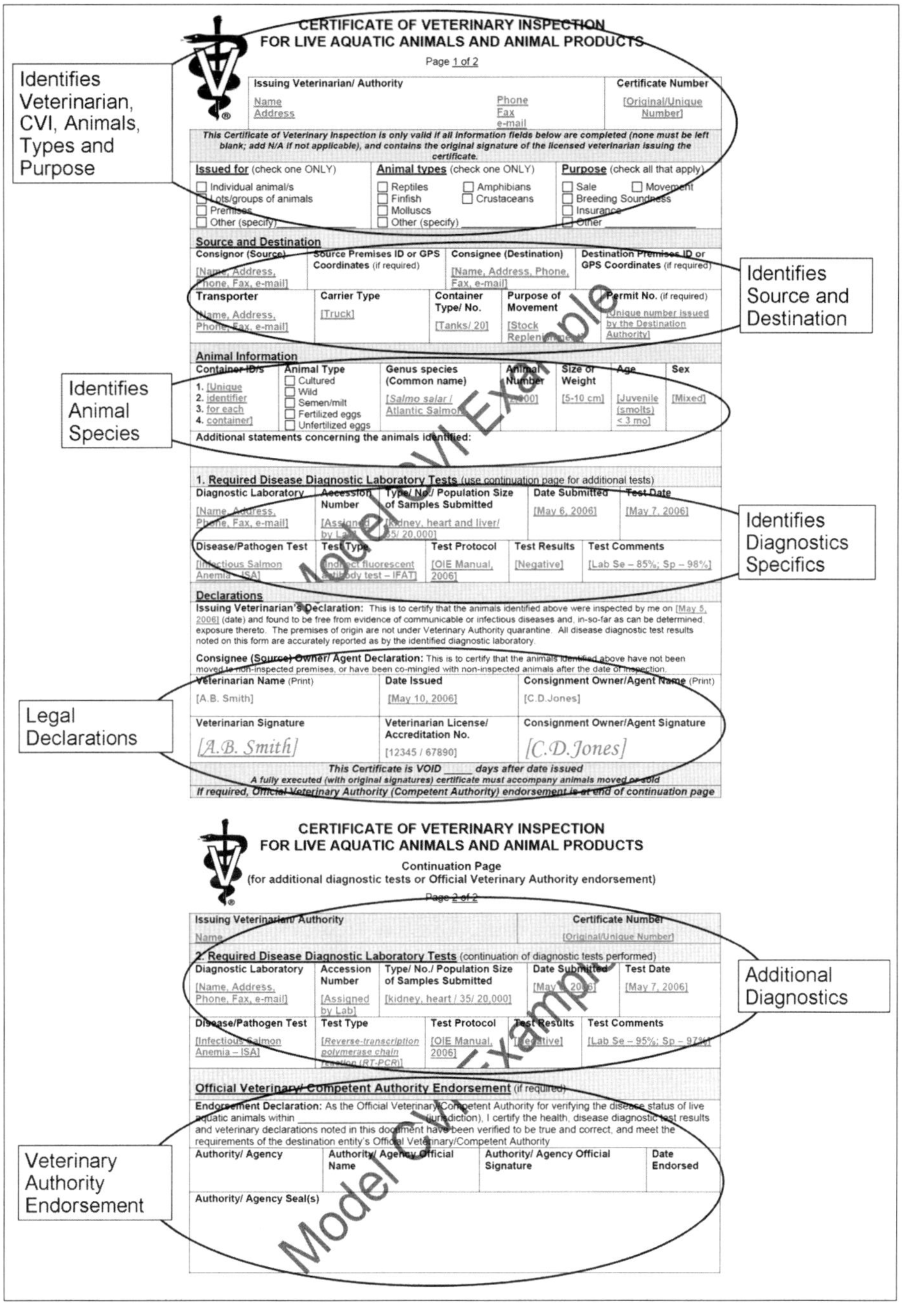

Fig. 1: A revised model aquatic CVI. This model CVI has broad potential use for individual operations, states or countries. It is produced for the purpose of illustration only. The sections of the CVI are discussed in the text.

Detailed information about the source and destination is provided in section 2. The origination ownership is recorded by name, address, telephone and other contact information. If the location of animal origination differs from the owner's contact information, additional information should be recorded for traceability of the animals such as place of origin address, contact information, GPS coordinates or other means of spatial identification. Information about how the animals are to be transported such as vehicle description/identification and any unique container identification along with the type and conditions of transport (number and type of containers) needs to be listed in section 2 of the CVI. The actual destination of the animals at time of unloading needs to be recorded in this section. Obviously, the receiving party's contact information should also be recorded if different than the animal destination location. Special permits (for example permit for the collection of wild animals, or truck driver animal handling permit) required by law or other regulations, or requested by the source/destination parties can also be listed in this section.

Detailed information to uniquely and specifically identify the animals subjected to the veterinary examination and sampled for laboratory submission is entered in section 3. The total number of animals, including identification numbers of the animals if individually tagged or marked, type of animals (cultured, wild captured, semen/milt, fertilized or unfertilized eggs), common and scientific species name, number, size, weight and sex of the animals are identified in this section.

The results of specific validated/standardized diagnostic tests required by the destination authority are listed in section 4. The information in this section is provided by the veterinarian or the competent authority and is based on the communication between the veterinarian and the laboratory personnel. Contact information about the laboratory (including accession number assigned to the sample by the laboratory), sample type (blood, tissue, whole animal) size, and dates need to be included, followed by the disease tested for, type of test performed and protocol followed. Laboratory test information recorded in this section should permit determination of the test's validity, and allow for calculation of the probability of disease/pathogen freedom [7,10]. The listing of the results of the test (positive/negative) is mandatory, but optional field(s) can be used to include additional information/comments about the test such as the veterinary practitioner's interpretation of the laboratory's results in the context of the observed conditions and facilities, at the time of examination, etc. Since more than one test may be required, this section of the CVI can be expanded with additional pages to include information on all performed tests.

Section 5 contains the legal declarations which have to be signed by the veterinarian attesting to adequate sampling, sample preparation, chain-of-custody of samples, observations of animals, facilities, conditions of care, and biosecurity procedures in place. The animal owner may also be required to attest to maintaining the animals in separate facilities and under quarantine until shipment or other release as advised by the practicing veterinarian. The time frame for which the CVI is valid has to be stated here, along with the statement that the fully executed (signed) CVI must accompany moved or sold animals.

In addition, to meet country requirements according to OIE standards [4], endorsement by the official veterinary authority (or other competent authority with jurisdiction over aquatic animal health) is provided as required by the importing country. This section has to be the last section of the document, and therefore listed on a continuation page, after additional diagnostic test information.

Future Progress for Increasing Efficiency: the Electronic CVI (e-CVI)

Existing and emerging foreign animal disease threats to today's animal industries indicate the need for real-time reports, prompt trace-back, immediate status notification and surveillance of aquatic and terrestrial animal health. Electronic health certificates offer an opportunity to incorporate the paper process into an electronic venue where disease monitoring and control of animal movement will safeguard animal health in general [11]. A secured electronic system in accord with OIE standards for the collection and transfer of data between the attending veterinarian, diagnostic laboratories, competent authorities and the source and destination, and for issuing e-CVIs would increase the utility of any CVI system (Fig. 2) [4]. The use of e-CVIs can provide potential benefits for state, federal and private veterinary practitioners, and animal health officials as well as animal industry producers and all trading partners. Furthermore, the opportunity for rapid tracking of animal origin, and movement, as well as readily available information associated with animal health status can increase emergency preparedness and response, allow for real time trace back and reports, and improve the early detection and surveillance of emerging diseases and identification of potential biosecurity threats [11,12].

A preliminary trial of an e-CVI system was successfully tested by GlobalVetLink (Ames, Iowa, USA) for moving 15-20 shipments of ornamental (aquarium) finfish per week (7-10,000 per shipment), from Florida wholesale sources to Virginia pet stores from 2001 to 2002 [5]. Currently, no system for issuing e-CVIs for aquatic animals is fully operational; however, several systems are in development such as GlobalVetLink's e-OCVI, and the United States Department of Agriculture Veterinary Services' Process Streamlining (USDA VSPS) (Fig. 3). The full implementation of the e-Interstate Certificate Veterinary Inspection in the VSPS program would be extremely useful and easily applicable for aquatic e-CVIs.

A similar approach would be feasible in the European Union by integrating TRACES (TRAde Control and Expert System), CENTAUR (database for export health certificates and transboundary animal disease e-communication) and ANIMO (computerized network for linking veterinary authorities) [13] or in Australia/New Zealand using a modified e-CERTS system (Fig 4).

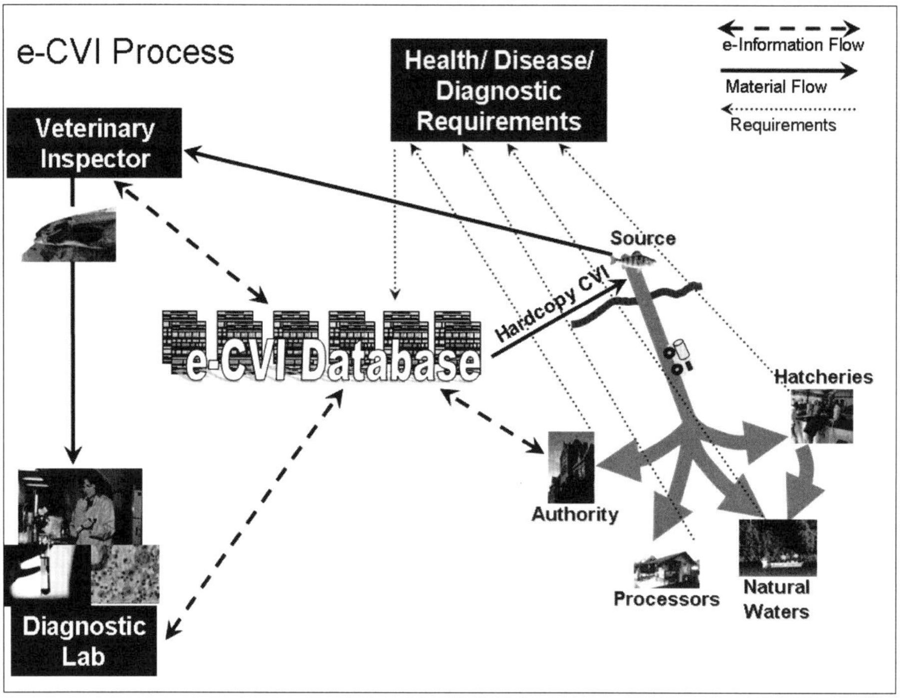

Fig. 2: The e-CVI process. A stylized example of how electronic information can be conveyed between individuals and entities (veterinarian, diagnostic laboratory, source and destination owners, and authorities, in developing an electronic Certificate of Veterinary Inspection.

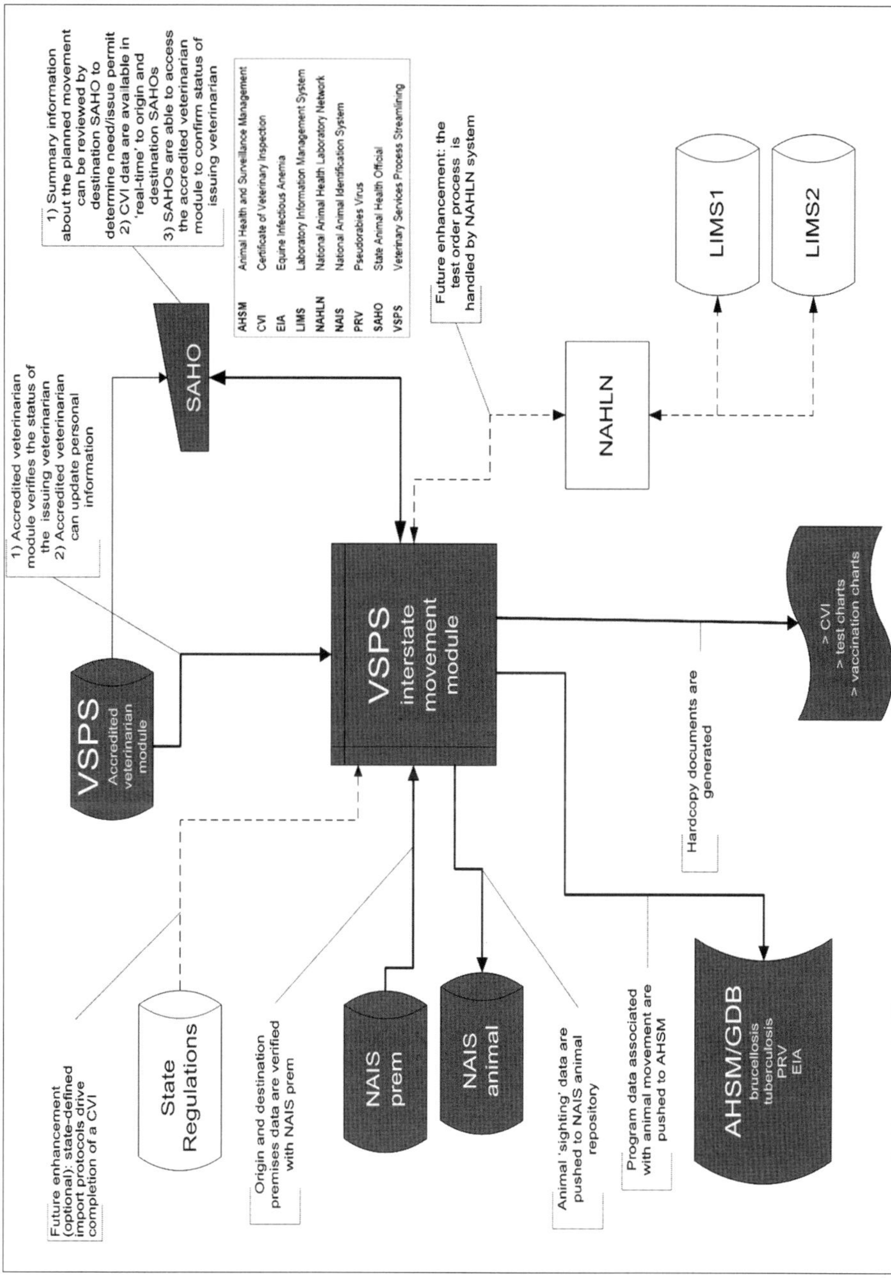

Fig. 3: USDA-APHIS "Veterinary Services Process Streamlining" (VSPS) concept. Under an "e-Government Initiative" (also developing in many other countries) the USDA Animal and Plant Health Inspection Service (APHIS) has proposed integrating multiple electronic data tracking and recording systems, including e-CVIs [11].

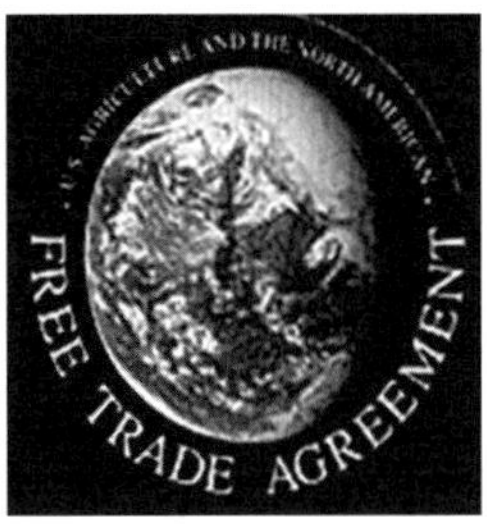

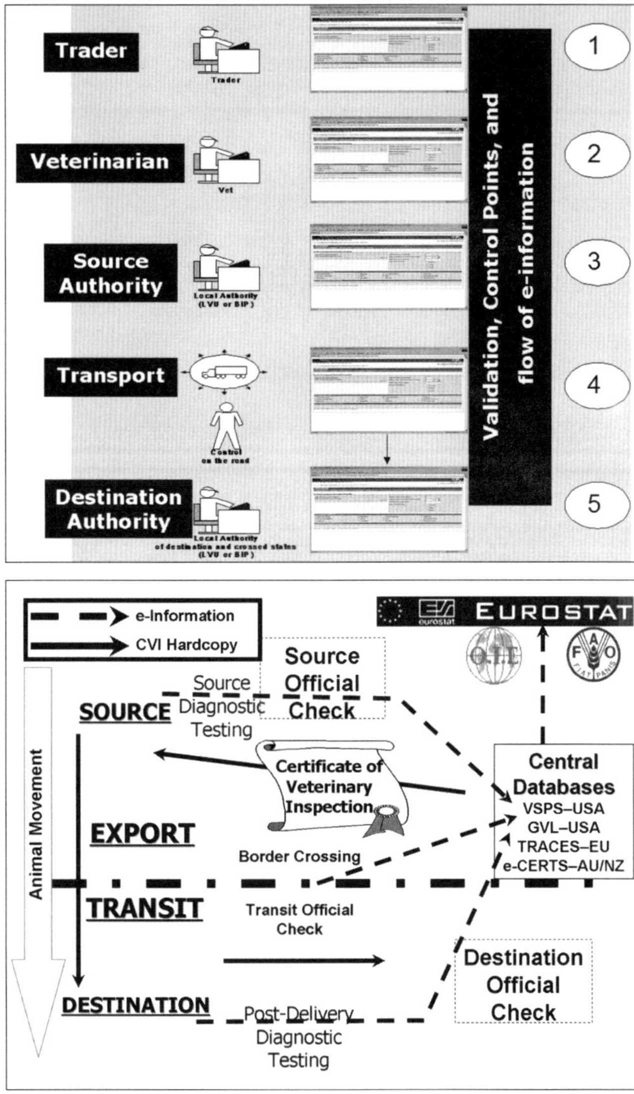

Fig. 4: e-CVI incorporation into "e-Government Initiatives". Schematic illustration of how systems may work to incorporate e-CVIs.

CONCLUSION

In accordance with the OIE Aquatic Animal Standards Commission Work Plan for 2006/2007 to reexamine "Health Certificates", these elements of a Certificate of Veterinary Inspection are offered for discussion, comment and refinement. The authors hope the thoughts proffered here will assist to simplify the veterinary certification processes for aquatic species; unify the processes with the time-proven terrestrial animal certification process; and enhance trade through universal uniformity. If optimally designed, model CVIs may be of use with electronic systems that are evolving in Europe, the USA and Australia/New Zealand in accord with governmental directives.

ACKNOWLEDGEMENTS

The authors thank many individuals from several organizations that have contributed to the development of concepts outlined here including: the American Veterinary Medical Association; the California Department of Fish and Game, the University of Florida, the Florida Tropical Aquaculture Laboratory, and the Florida Department of Agriculture and Consumer Services; GlobalVetLink, L.C.; the Maine Departments of Agriculture and Inland Fisheries and Wildlife; the National Association of State Aquaculture Coordinators; the Wisconsin Department of Agriculture, Trade & Consumer Protection; USDA, and the Center for Epidemiology and Animal Health.

REFERENCES

1. Hill BJ: The Need for Effective Disease Control in International Aquaculture. Midtlyng PJ (ed): Progress in Fish Vaccinology, Dev Biol (Basel) 2005;121:3-12.
2. FAO: State of World Aquaculture, FAO Fisheries Technical Paper No 500, FAO, Rome, 2006.
3. Daszak P, Cunningham AA, Hyatt AD: Emerging Infectious Diseases of Wildlife: Threats to Biodiversity and Human Health. Science 2000;287:443-49.
4. OIE: Aquatic Animal Code Certification Procedures: Electronic Certification, World Organisation for Animal Health, Paris, 2006, 27.
5. Scarfe AD: Electronic Certificates of Veterinary Inspection (e-CVI) – A Model Health Assurance Program for U.S. Aquaculture Industries. Proceedings of the International Association for Aquatic Animal Medicine, 2004, Galveston, Texas, April 4-8.
6. ODA: Certificate of Veterinary Inspection, O. D. o. Agriculture, Oregon Department of Agriculture, 2006
7. OIE: Manual of Diagnostic Tests for Aquatic Animals, World Organization for Animal Health, Paris, 2006.
8. Scarfe AD: Aquatic veterinary education, training and credentials supporting animal health and diseases programs. OIE Global Conference on Aquatic Animal Health, 2006, Bergen, Norway.
9. Session V: Education and Training Needs in Aquatic Animal Health. In: Dodet B, the OIE Scientific & Technical Department (eds): The OIE Global Conference on Aquatic Animal Health. Dev Biol (Basel). Basel, Karger, 2007; 129:93-146.
10. Cameron A: Survey Toolbox for Aquatic Animal Diseases: A Practical Manual and Software Package, Australian Centre for International Research, Canberra, 2002, p 375.
11. APHIS: Veterinary Services Process Streamlining, United States Department of Agriculture Animal and Plant Health Inspection Service, 2006.

12. Cummings D: VSPS e-Interstate Module: e-CVI Setting the Gold Standard. U.S. Animal Health Association Annual Meeting, 2005, Greensboro, SC, USA. October 21-27.

13. TRACES, CENTAUR and ANIMO: are currently being examined in response to several EU Council Directives (e.g. 89/662/EEC, 90/425/EEC, 91/496/EEC, 97/78/EC, and others), 2006, http://europa.eu.int/eur-lex/

Dr. David Scarfe, AVMA, PO Box 6100, Mississippi States, MS 39762, USA
E-mail: David Scarfe: DScarfe@avma.org

Dodet B, the OIE Scientific & Technical Department (eds): The OIE Global Conference on Aquatic Animal Health. Dev Biol (Basel). Basel, Karger, 2007, vol 129, p 103.

Session V

Education and Training Needs in Aquatic Animal Health

Chairperson: *R. Enriquez*, Chile

Dodet B, the OIE Scientific & Technical Department (eds): The OIE Global Conference on Aquatic Animal Health. Dev Biol (Basel). Basel, Karger, 2007, vol 129, pp 105-113.

Experiences in Providing Training and Education in Aquatic Animal Health

L. Pollock, R. Richards

Institute of Aquaculture, University of Stirling, Stirling, UK

Key words: training, aquatic animal health, Institute of Aquaculture, courses

Abstract: The Institute of Aquaculture brings together cross-disciplinary researchers to meet the wide range of training challenges faced as the global aquaculture industry grows. The Institute offers training in a range of academic levels from short courses, aimed at farm operatives, to BSc (Hons), MSc and PhD levels. The focus of training at the Institute is on promoting a holistic approach, emphasising the importance of understanding the aquatic production system as a whole as well as detailed knowledge of specific pathogens. To make training more accessible, the Institute has made the provision of Continuing Professional Development (CPD) a strategic objective and provides distance learning and flexible study options.

INTRODUCTION

The Institute of Aquaculture was established in 1971 as the Unit of Aquatic Pathology. As the aquaculture industry grew, the unit developed into the Institute of Aquaculture covering the broad range of aquaculture-related sciences it does today.

The Institute of Aquaculture initially focused on servicing the needs of the established British trout production industry and fish health issues present in wild fish populations. During the pioneering stages of the salmon industry in the 1980s, it expanded to service the requirement for both research and training critical for the industry's development. The Institute increased its capacity in the aquatic animal health field, but also began to increase the range of specialist areas required to support sustainable sector growth. The research areas grew to include a number of species including tilapia and carp in Asia and Mediterranean sea bass and sea bream.

Graded 5 in the 2001 Research Assessment Exercise (RAE) of the Higher Education Funding Council (HEFC) of the UK, the Institute now brings together cross-disciplinary researchers to meet the wide range of challenges faced as aquaculture grows to meet global demands. Research focuses on questions relating to strategies for sustainable aquaculture, whether for modern commercial markets or for feeding poor communities in developing countries. Fundamental research on environments, reproduction, genetics, aquatic health, nutrition and feed supplies, production systems, markets, and social and economic impacts continues to play significant roles. The Institute has grown steadily over the last 35 years and now employs more than 110 staff and has 120 postgraduate students.

The Need for Training in Aquatic Animal Health

Due to expansion and intensification, the global aquaculture sector has grown at an average rate of 8.8 percent per year since 1970, compared with only 1.2 percent for capture fisheries and 2.8 percent in 2004 for terrestrial farmed meat production systems over the same period. Production in 2004 was reported to have risen to 59.4 million tonnes, with a value of 70.3 billion $US [1], highlighting that the economic value of aquaculture is large and increasing.

As aquaculture continues to expand and intensify, aquatic animal diseases have the opportunity to emerge and cause devastating losses to both industrial and small-scale producers.

Disease is now a significant constraint to production in intensive systems and causes the loss of aquatic animal production through sub-optimal growth and mortality. The movement of seed and broodstock has been pivotal in the potential for pathogen introduction. Translocation of pathogens through the increase in movement and trade in live aquatic species and aquatic products triggered by the internationalisation of markets has accelerated the spread of diseases [2].

The risk of disease is enough to reduce investor confidence and has been linked to the lack of Government supported compensatory measures [3]. Such losses in investor confidence can have a devastating impact on aquaculture production. As the global population continues to grow, food production systems must both expand and intensify to meet demand, therefore any disease crisis affecting production and/or market prices will have a considerable impact on both producers, service and input providers and consumers.

In this context, the need for specialised education in both aquaculture management and aquatic animal health is necessary to ensure good aquatic animal welfare and sustainable production.

Teaching Aquatic Animal Health Management – The Approach

"How does one define disease - the presence of lesions - loss of production biomass, poor nutritional status - inherited genetic traits - malformations and stress?"

Gaining an overall understanding of the production system in order to understand the relationship between the role of stressors in aquatic animal rearing systems and pathogens themselves is critical to fully understand the status of aquatic animal health. In aquatic animal production systems there are strong linkages between an animal's biology, environment, nutrition, genetic origin and its health.

The prevalence of non-infectious diseases becomes increasingly apparent in intensive culture systems. The impact of stocking density, water flow rates, and genetic or nutritional factors can impact on health. Examples of this include spinal deformities or cataracts caused by histidine deficiency in diets lacking bloodmeal. Clearly, disease manifests itself in a number of ways and causative factors can only be fully understood by looking at the culture system, its inputs and its practices in concurrence with the suspected pathogens themselves. The Institute of Aquaculture places an emphasis on understanding the pathogen, environment and host interactions in its teaching approach.

Programmes of Study

The Institute has successfully run courses for fish farmers since 1973. Today, training is offered in a range of academic levels from short courses, aimed at farm operatives, to BSc (Hons), MSc and PhD levels. The undergraduate BSc degree in aquaculture provides an overview of all aspects of aquatic animal and plant culture. Some training in disease is introduced at this level. The majority of detailed aquatic animal health training occurs at the MSc level, where specialist Masters degrees can be taken in Aquatic Veterinary Studies or Aquatic Pathobiology.

In human health contexts, understanding lifestyle is a critical feature of understanding where disease may occur, and if it does, how to manage it. The same is true for aquatic animal health. A good aquatic animal health specialist will have a fundamental understanding of aquatic animal production systems as well as the ability to identify and manage specific pathogens. The Institute's teaching places a significant emphasis on understanding aquatic animal husbandry practice in conjunction with the study of aquatic animal pathology and pathogen identification methods. Analytical techniques are also taught in fields such as histopathology, immunology technologies, molecular techniques such as proteomics and genomics; however, the results of these analyses require careful interpretation, taking into account the wider context. A solid grounding in aquatic animal production systems, biology, nutrition, genetics, reproduction and environment is emphasised in all aquatic animal health training at the Institute of Aquaculture, with the principal aim of enabling candidates to reach well informed diagnoses.

An overview of aquatic animal biology is given with the emphasis placed on satifying the physiological and biological requirements of aquatic animals in the culture environment. This is followed by an introduction to the main viral, parasitic and fungal diseases of fish and shrimp and their diagnosis and treatment. Practical sampling sessions and case studies are used at this stage, allowing for the early introduction of hands-on work for those with no previous aquaculture or aquatic animal health experience.

Understanding aquatic animals and their relationship with the environment is also vital to understanding their health. This course module on environment takes into account aquatic physio-chemical processes, and community structure and function. There are two field sessions within the module including a freshwater and marine site visit with practical sampling sessions at each. Environmental risk assessment and the environmental impacts of aquaculture are key components.

Nutrition is also a vital element of aquatic animal health. The nutrition module aids understanding of the principles of aquatic animal nutrition. This module covers the major nutritional needs of aquatic animals and feeding needs over a number of different aquaculture systems ranging from extensive and semi-intensive pond systems to intensive re-circulating and cage aquaculture systems in both temperate and tropical climes. There is also considerable discussion of feed formulation, manufacture and practical husbandry, providing relevant background.

The aquatic animal genetics and reproduction module creates the opportunity to learn about broodstock management, spawning, egg quality and gender control using a series of lectures and practical sessions. The application of genetic manipulation in aquaculture includes hybridisation, sex reversal, quantitative genetics and cryopreservation. The module covers a number of the most commercially important species such as salmon, rainbow trout, cod, halibut, carp and tilapia. There is strong emphasis on hatchery processes including larval rearing, hatchery operation, design and management.

The production systems themselves are explored in a module which covers a wide range of aquaculture production systems and includes consideration of system design for both land and water based systems of many aquatic species. The production system is explored from the hatchery through to grow-out. Engineering components across pond, tank and cage and recirculation systems, taking into account water treatment are discussed.

As exposure to the principles of aquaculture is established, a study tour of aquaculture operations is taken to establish the necessary field experience.

By the end of this phase, students should be able to appraise a number of aquaculture systems for a number of species and be able to make the link between the processes of aquatic animal production, husbandry practice and aquatic animal health.

Specialist Understanding of Diseases

Following an overview of aquatic animal production systems and the processes therein, a number of specialist pathogens and pathogen identification methods are covered through modules in systemic pathology and histopathology, parasitology, immunology, microbial diseases, ecotoxicology, health management and epidemiology.

Systemic pathology and histopathology is taught through a series of practical sessions, enabling students to develop core competencies in the area and experience some of the practical diagnostic work at the Institute. This module aims to allow students to identify and describe a wide range of histopathological changes and arrive at a histopathological diagnosis of the more common conditions, including suggested aetiology and treatment.

Parasitology is a major area of expertise and training in this area and the parasitology module ensures a basic knowledge of the wide variety of parasitic fish pathogens. Sufficient knowledge of their taxonomy, morphology and lifecycle strategies is delivered to identify pathogens in both aquaculture and fisheries in temperate and tropical, marine and freshwater environments. Special attention is also given to current problems, especially where there is a significant economic impact. Throughout the module, issues of stock and parasite management and control are emphasised.

Immunology teaching focuses on the biochemical means of detecting viral problems in fish. A large practical element of the course uses techniques such as ELISA and immunohistochemistry to monitor immune responses in fish following exposure to infection or vaccine. The identification of vaccine antigens using electrophoresis and Western blotting is also covered to enable students to gain an understanding of fish immunology and its application for vaccine development, the use of antibody probes in fish health control, fish vaccine development and administration, and the advantages and disadvantages of various immunological methods versus traditional diagnostic methods.

Training in microbial diseases has a strong focus on the principles of microbiology and trains students on the techniques of isolating and identifying a number of aquatic animal pathogens including viruses, bacteria and mycological pathogens.

As a number of chemotherapeutants are used in aquaculture, training in ecotoxicology is important to cover toxicological and ecological assessments. This module offers an understanding of the principles governing toxicity of pollutants in living organisms in the major classes of chemical pollutants and investigates their environmental fate, the major aquaculture chemotherapeutants and their ecotoxicity, the use of biomarkers in ecotoxicology and the use of new molecular technologies as applied to ecotoxicology.

The emphasis on epidemiology in aquatic animal health training aims to formalise the instinctive process of looking for patterns in disease situations in order to gain an overview of the progression of a disease situation. Epidemiological principals are followed by population sampling exercises such as sample size calculation and analysis of outbreak information. This information is synthesised to enable differential diagnoses to be developed. Understanding of risk factors and means of controlling suspected disease outbreaks are critical elements of the taught programmes. Current issues for which training in epidemiology is useful include the control and treatment of sea lice – when to treat, treatment rotation, the impact on and effect of wild fish and the management of *Gyrodactylus salaries*, how to keep it out and what to do if it enters the UK.

Difference in Focus

The needs of the aquaculture industry tend to centre around husbandry issues: guidance on what can be done to prevent disease, the rapid diagnosis of disease, and appropriate treatment to save stocks and mitigate economic losses. Professional training is needed as the aquaculture industry becomes increasingly governed by codes of practice, such as the Code of Good Practice for Scottish Finfish Aquaculture [4].

Official controls have often taken an emphasis on sensitive and specific pathogen identification tests. However, there is also a need for those involved in the regulatory sector to take a balanced overview of containment measures and a need for more modelling and strategic planning. Training is also available for official governmental fish health inspectors to allow for better understanding of the requirements of the aquaculture production industry.

New Developments in Training Delivery

Increasing emphasis on animal welfare

The Council of Europe has drafted recommendations on the welfare of fish which may be used as the basis for a European Directive. The industry is showing an increase in interest in welfare aspects of farmed fish production. Consumer awareness of food production systems and the proliferation of food labelling schemes are also growing and it is likely that in the future, producers will need to demonstrate to retailers that the basic welfare standards of their farmed fish have been met throughout the production cycle. In view of this emerging area, there is now an emphasis on aquatic animal welfare within the MSc programmes at the Institute of Aquaculture.

Professional standards

There is an increasing need for the recognition of professional competencies within many professional bodies including the veterinary profession. The need for Continuing Professional Development (CPD) and has led to a demand from regulatory bodies to provide training in aquatic animal health to their key staff. The Institute of Aquaculture has made the provision of CPD a strategic objective. The modularisation of programmes facilitating this objective has proven to be successful in attracting participants from the commercial sector seeking specialist career development training.

Distance learning provision

There is an increasing demand for CPD in order for employees to stay abreast of the latest developments in their field. However, opportunities for study are often limited by the demands of full-time employment, travel and/or family commitments. Hence, there is a need for more flexible means of delivering quality CPD training. A recent initiative by the Institute of Aquaculture has culminated in the development of a PG Certificate in Aquatic Animal Health, which aims to meet professional training requirements whilst allowing participants to maintain their current work-life balance.

The aim of the PG Certificate programme is to recognise and standardise professional competence for those working within the field of aquatic animal health.

The programme aims to train participants in the disciplines apposite to investigation, prevention and control of disease in the marine and freshwater environment. Although the programme was principally developed to meet the needs of those in a regulatory role, it is also of relevance to anyone with professional involvement in aquatic animal health, in a veterinary, production or regulatory role.

The programme delivers training on a part-time basis using a mix of web-based and practical learning. The programme structure is comprised of six modules which are taken over a period of three years. These modules cover areas including fish biology, health and epidemiology, aquatic environments, aquaculture nutrition, aquaculture genetics, reproduction and systemic pathology and histopathology. The programme aims to develop a systems approach to first establishing a differential diagnosis and then progressing to a definitive diagnosis. This is assessed with a final diagnostic case study through which the candidates must demonstrate their ability to draw on all their knowledge of husbandry and specific diseases.

Flexible study

A move towards more flexible study has made it possible for all face-to-face taught postgraduate programmes to be delivered on a full-time or a discontinuous basis. This new approach has been developed to fit the needs of those currently with employment and/or with family commitments that limit their time to study for further career development. This flexible approach to training is designed to fit around the lifestyles of those working in aquaculture, particularly rural workers, who want to learn but can't afford to take time out for longer periods of study.

Programmes are modularised into two week blocks. This enables a discontinuous study mode where students may attend a module for two weeks and then break their study to return to work. Credits for each module taken are accumulated towards a postgraduate qualification. CPD candidates may also wish to attend single modules purely for professional training or interest. This is also possible. Furthermore, the Institute of Aquaculture has increased the time period for completion of a postgraduate qualification from three years to a maximum of five years to facilitate this path.

Widening Access to Education

Recognising that not all those involved in aquaculture and fish health have formal qualifications, the University accepts that the possession of standard entry qualifications is not in itself evidence of incapacity to undertake higher education. A person's work experience can now be credited through the University of Stirling in order to gain entry to some academic programmes. A quality assurance procedure has been developed for this function and candidates' experience is assessed against a number of criteria which take into account the level and volume of such experience and its appropriateness for the qualification sought.

In recognition of the fact that not all those involved in aquatic animal health wish to formalise their professional training with an academic award, the Institute of Aquaculture allows candidates to attend each of their academic modules without assessment in a non-credit bearing mode.

Assessments cover a range of learning styles throughout the programme and included techniques for those who learn visually, orally, through reading and writing, or use kinaesthetic (learning through experience or practice) learning styles. Most people are multimodal in their learning styles and a range of assessment types can suit them. However, by varying the nature of activities and assessments to test a range of learning outcomes, those with stronger learning preferences may also be accommodated.

The Institute also continues to run its Fish Health short course and other specialist short courses aimed at those working within the aquaculture industry at both farm operative and managerial levels, and it continues to attract substantial interest.

Conclusion

The experiences of the Institute of Aquaculture in delivering training in aquatic animal health have shown that education must be provided in a different way. People are limited by time and wish to complete education in the most flexible, cost effective and convenient way for them. Increasingly, this means remaining employed whilst undertaking some form of study.

The introduction of professional standards and the need for industry and regulators to implement employee CPD programmes has driven a change in the way training is delivered at the Institute of Aquaculture. We are increasing our distance and blended learning provision in a move to promote more flexible study arrangements.

Despite the changes in delivery, the focus of the Institute remains the same. It continues to promote a holistic approach, emphasising the importance of understanding the aquatic production system as a whole as well as detailed knowledge of specific pathogens.

References

1 FAO: The State of the World Fisheries and Aquaculture 2006. Food and Agriculture Organisation of the United Nations, Rome, 2007.

2 Subasinghe RR, Bontad-Reantaso MG, McGladdery SE: Aquaculture development, health and wealth, in: Subasinghe RP, Bueno P, Phillips MJ, Hough C, McGladdery SE, Arthur JR (eds.): Aquaculture in the Next Millennium. Technical Proceedings of the Conference on Aquaculture in the Third Millennium, Bangkok, Thailand, 20-25 February 2000. NACA, Bangkok and FAO, Rome, 2001, pp167 - 191.

3 Scottish Executive: Aquaculture and Fisheries Bill. Consultation Paper and Draft Regulatory Impact Assessment, 2005, Annex A., Part 5, Item 65http://www.scotland.gov.uk/Publications /2005/12/1494325/43302, Date of access: April 2007.

4 Scottish Fin Fish Aquaculture Working Group: Code of Good Practice for Fin Fish Producers, 2007, http://www.scottishsalmon.co.uk/dlDocs/CoGp.pdf, Date of Access: 12th April 2007.

Pr. Randolph H. Richards, Institute of Aquaculture, University of Stirling, Stirling FK9 4LA, Scotland, UK
E-mail: r.h.richards@stir.ac.uk

Dodet B, the OIE Scientific & Technical Department (eds): The OIE Global Conference on Aquatic Animal Health. Dev Biol (Basel). Basel, Karger, 2007, vol 129, pp 115-123.

PANDA Assessment of Needs and Training Opportunities in Aquatic Animal Health

M. Hiney

National University of Ireland Galway, Galway City, Ireland

Key words: PANDA project, training, aquatic animal health, Europe

Abstract: A survey on training needs and opportunities among aquatic animal health professionals was carried out as part of the EU funded PANDA project. A preliminary analysis of the data revealed that in terms of training participation, over 65% of responders had participated in training within the previous six months and that this training consisted predominantly of short courses or conferences. However, 20% of responders had not participated in training in the previous three or more years, with time and money being the major reasons cited for non-participation. Occupation and location in Europe would also appear to have an impact on frequency of training and on the type of training undertaken. Responders' own organisations played a key role in training provision, while international training bodies constituted an important source of applied training. Universities did not play an important role in training. In terms of training needs, newer diagnostic methods for bacterial and viral diseases were the principle training needs identified. Epidemiology and risk analysis were also identified as training needs that are not currently fulfilled. The majority of responders felt that the EU should have more involvement in training provision and formulation of policy around training.

This paper was not presented orally, as scheduled, as Dr. Hiney was unable to attend the conference.

Introduction

In 2005, as part of the EU funded PANDA Concerted Action project, a survey on training opportunities and deficits in aquatic animal disease research and diagnosis was undertaken among people involved in the broad area of fish heath management. The survey focused on training in disease diagnosis, method validation and quality assurance, epidemiology, risk analysis and environmentally sustainable practices. The objectives of the survey were to: identify current levels of participation in training opportunities; identify primary delivery methods for training; seek stakeholder experience on the utility of, and access to, training (both for themselves and other stakeholder groups); and seek information on stakeholder experience regarding current training deficits.

The survey took the form of a comprehensive questionnaire that covered the following sections: demography of respondents, frequency and type of training undertaken, training providers and information sources, reasons for not participating in training and factors that might facilitate training, and the impact of EU involvement in training policy and provision. The results of this survey will form part of a broader recommendation document to the European Commission at the completion of the PANDA project in 2007.

Materials and Methods

A draft version of the questionnaire was piloted with a group of 14 scientists at the National Reference Laboratory meeting in Aarhus, in June 2005. Sections of the questionnaire were revised to reflect the feedback of the pilot group regarding ease of use, duplication, appropriateness of questions etc. In order to achieve a wide distribution of the questionnaire among a variety of stakeholders (scientists, regulators, practitioners, fisheries biologists, etc.), a web-based survey tool (WebSurveyor) was tested with regard to ease of data input and data handling, extraction and analysis. In particular, ease of use by respondents was considered critical to achieving a good response rate; where possible drop-down lists and tick boxes, etc., were used.

An e-mail distribution list was constructed from a number of electronic and paper-based sources (EAFP Members' Handbook, Coordinator's personal list etc.). E-mail addresses from the USA, Canada, South America, Asia and Australia were omitted, because this survey was intended to look at the European situation. The survey was also distributed via the PANDA subscribers mailing list, the AquaTT mailing list, the University of Stirling mailing list and the mailing lists of the Regional Reference Laboratories for both fish and shellfish diseases. Approximately 4,000 people received the survey from these distributions lists. Surveys with 10 or more questions completed, out of 20 questions posed, were considered to be valid.

RESULTS

Demographic information

There were a total of 281 valid responses from all over Europe. With duplicate postings taken into account this represents a response rate of approximately 12.5%, which is in line with the expected response rate for surveys of this type. Responses were received, in order of number, from researchers and regulatory personnel, aquaculture and allied services companies and professional associations. For the purposes of data analysis, Europe was divided into four geographical, as opposed to political, regions: Northern, Western, Eastern and Southern Europe.

Table 1: Respondents by European Country

Region	Country	No. of Valid Responses
Southern Europe	Malta	1
	Turkey	3
	Portugal	8
	Greece	8
	Italy	11
	Spain	32
Northern Europe	Sweden	1
	Iceland	4
	Finland	10
	Denmark	13
	Norway	18
Western Europe	Switzerland	2
	Austria	3
	Belgium	4
	Netherlands	5
	Germany	9
	France	11
	Ireland	14
	UK	38
Eastern Europe	Poland	1
	Croatia	1
	Czech Republic	1
	Estonia	1
	Hungary	1
	Russia	1
	Slovakia	1
	Lithuania	2
	Romania	3
	Slovenia	3

The response rate from the countries within each region is shown in Table 1. In terms of occupation, there was a representative spread of the occupations associated with fish health management. The majority of respondents identified themselves as scientists, veterinarians, graduate students and government agency and regulatory personnel, while there was a smaller number of laboratory and aquaculture technicians, field biologists, fish farmers and specialist consultants. In light of the distribution lists employed, it was not surprising that the majority of respondents worked in universities, research institutions, fisheries research services and government laboratories, while a smaller number worked with aquaculture companies or professional associations.

Training participation

Over 65% of responders had participated in training in the previous year, with the majority (2/3) having done so within the previous six months. However, 20% of respondents had not participated in training within three or more years of completing the survey (Figure 1). Technical staff, fish farmers, and regulatory personnel were less likely to have participated in training within the previous two years while administrators, agency scientists, field biologists, graduate students and veterinarians were more likely to have participated in training in the previous two years. Interestingly, 43% of regulatory personnel who completed the survey had not participated in any kind of training within the previous three years. Respondents were also less likely to have participated in training within the previous three years if they were located in Eastern European countries.

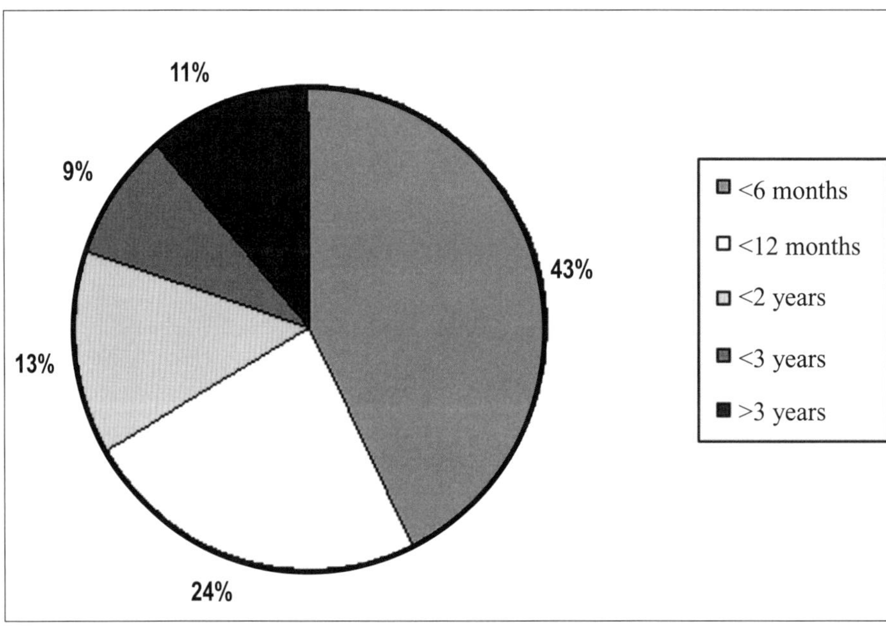

Fig. 1: Pie chart indicating the last time respondents undertook training

Figure 2 details the reasons respondents gave for not participating in training. Time and money were the major reasons cited, although lack of information or the unavailability of suitable courses was also considered important impediments to training. Lack of funding and the difficulties this posed in travelling outside their area were key impediments to training identified by respondents in Southern European countries, while lack of time was considered a greater impediment to training in Western Europe.

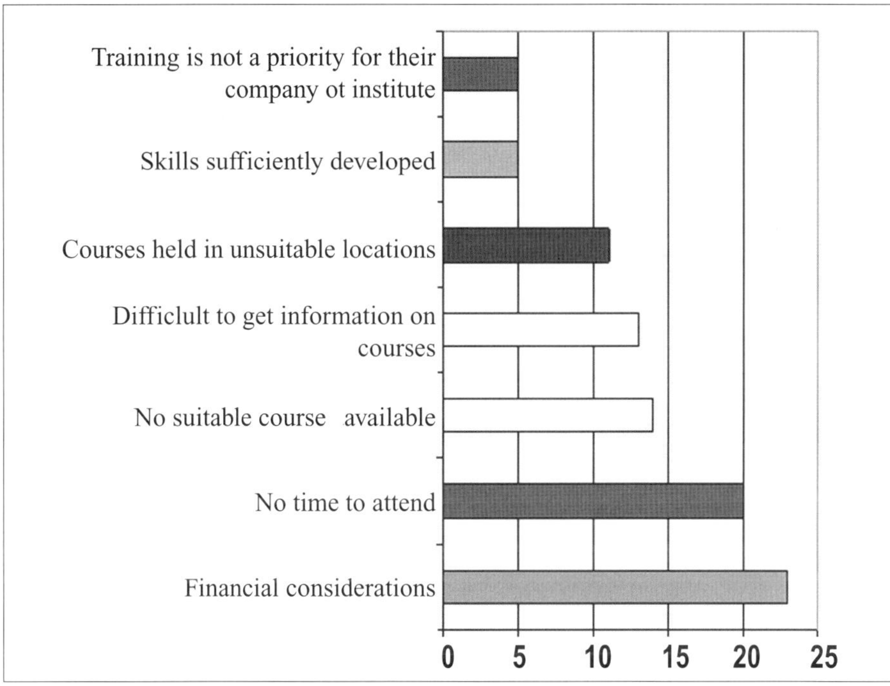

Fig. 2: Reasons given for not participating in training

Type of training undertaken

The type of training undertaken was generally compatible with the occupation of responders and included disease diagnostic methods (laboratory and field), general laboratory methods, specific courses in aquatic animal health and to a lesser extent, laboratory and field QA, and regulatory control (Figure 3). The least amount of training was undertaken in epidemiology/risk analysis. In addition, respondents located in Eastern European countries were less likely to undertake training in diagnostic methods than other Europeans and more likely to undertake training in laboratory QA than their colleagues elsewhere.

Provision of training

Training was predominantly of short duration and was either in the form of a conference or workshop. Responders' own organisations played a key role in providing training in all topics. International training bodies (e.g. AquaTT) constituted an important source of applied training, especially in Northern and Southern European countries, while national training bodies were more active in this role in Western European countries. Professional Associations were also identified as playing a role in applied training provision, especially in Northern and Eastern European countries. Word of mouth and e-mail accounted for almost 50% of information dissemination about training events, while newspaper and magazine advertisements had little impact on dissemination of training information (Figure 4).

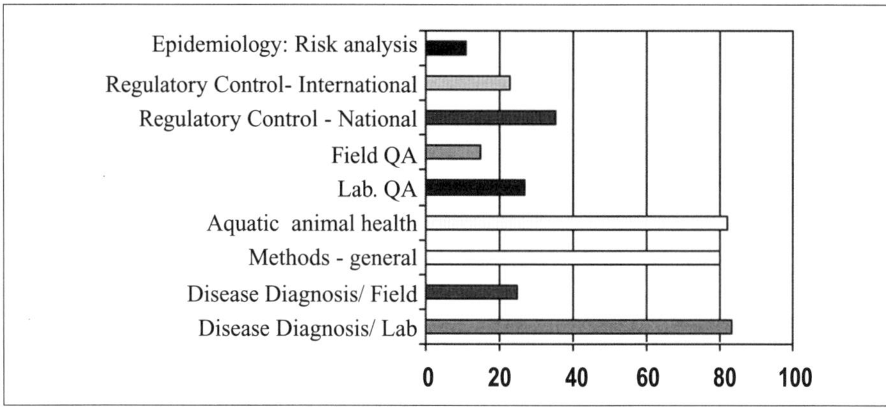

Fig. 3: Type of training undertaken by respondents in the previous three years

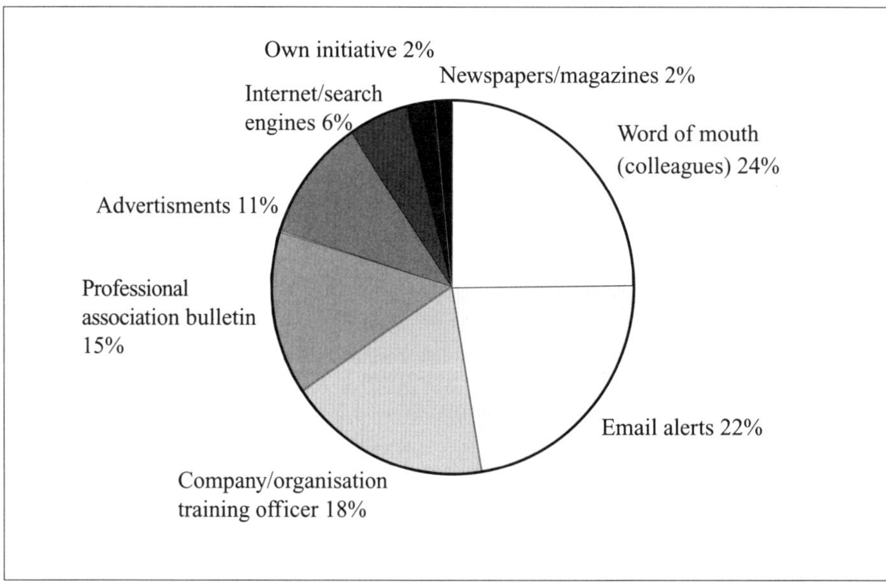

Fig. 4: Sources of training information used by survey respondents

Training needs

Figure 5 summarises the desired additional training identified by respondents. Diagnostic methods for bacteria and viruses (especially newer molecular methods) were the principle training needs identified. Epidemiology and risk analysis was also identified as training needs that are not being serviced at the moment. For aquaculture workers, field diagnosis and fish health management were the key training topics identified, while for veterinarians and other field specialists disease diagnosis and eradication methods were a key topic identified. Very few respondents overall were interested in, or felt the need for, training in quality assurance, regulatory issues or surveillance methods. When questioned about their knowledge of where their desired training might be provided, over 50% of respondents did not know where to look for the training they needed. The major elements determined as facilitators of training echoed to some extent the reasons cited for not undertaking training; respondents felt that availability of funding, specialist workshops and better information on training opportunities would best facilitate their participation in training activities.

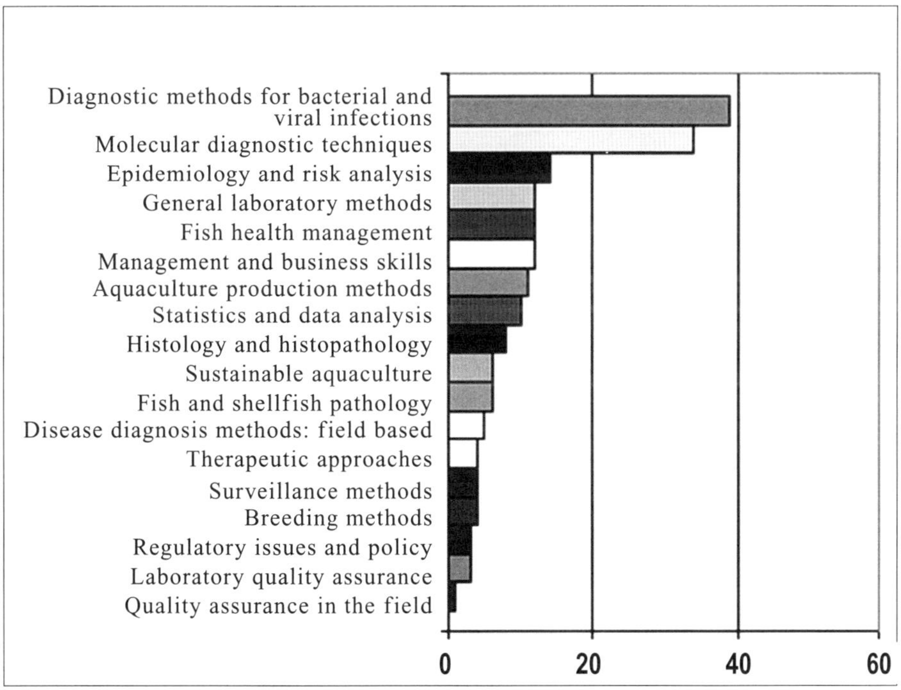

Fig. 5: Desired additional training identified by respondents

EU involvement in training policy and provision

The majority of responders felt that the European Commission (EC) should have more involvement in training provision and formulation of policy around training and identified a number of benefits from both. In terms of both policy formulation and training provision, the benefits of EC involvement were considered to be better harmonisation of standards across Europe leading to improved fish health management, more harmonisation of regulations and policies across Europe, coordinated use of diagnostic and control methods, improved quality assurance and ultimately improved product quality. Some respondents also felt that EC involvement in policy formulation would lead to better awareness of current and developing problems and improved dissemination of information on those problems. In addition to these benefits, respondents also expressed the opinion that provision of training by the EC would result in improvement of the skills base across Europe and provide a better funding base for training provision, which would be more focused and cost effective.

Discussion

While a response rate of 12.5% might be normal for a survey of this type, it nonetheless constrains the conclusions that can be drawn from the survey. In addition, the use of a web-based survey may have introduced bias by targeting only those who are both computer literate and have regular access to e-mail. That said, the survey does raise some interesting issues regarding the type, frequency and availability of training undertaken and desired by those engaged in fish health management across Europe.

On-going professional training was clearly important for respondents working in a laboratory setting (agency and laboratory scientists, laboratory technicians and graduate students, and veterinarians) and reflects a need to keep abreast of the latest developments in disease diagnostic methods and emerging or re-emerging disease problems. However, in some instances (10%) respondents commented that their training needs were quite specialised and that relevant training was unavailable to them or difficult to locate within Europe. The low number of respondents in this group who undertook training in laboratory QA might reflect the QA structures in place in many institutes and universities, where responsibility for compliance is given to a QA specialist, and is not considered a necessary part of the skills-base for laboratory workers. Laboratory and Field QA training were more likely to have been undertaken by respondents from Eastern European countries, perhaps reflecting monitoring and diagnostic laboratory structures in those countries that are still in the development phase.

It might be expected that personnel working in the field (field biologists, aquaculture technicians, consultants, fish farmers) would be less likely to participate in frequent training. Nonetheless, respondents felt that training of aquaculture workers and field biologists was essential, especially in the areas of fish health management and preliminary disease diagnosis. When asked who might provide this training, respondents indicated that professional associations, national and international training bodies, and to a lesser extent aquaculture companies, should do this. Universities were not seen to have an important role in provision of training to these stakeholders. A surprising result from the survey was the number of regulatory personnel who reported that they had not participated in any kind of training within the past three years. It was not clear from the survey why this might be the case.

The identified impediments to participation in training appear to be influenced by geographical area. In Southern European countries a lack of funding and travel to training locations outside the geographical area were identified as major impediments while in Northern and Western European countries lack of time and the unavailability of specialist courses were key. Interestingly, a sizable percentage of Western European respondents indicated that training was not a priority for their institutions or that their skills were sufficiently developed already. Where training was undertaken, it tended to be a workshop, symposium or seminar, held as part of a conference (67.8% of respondents). This would suggest that more 'add-on' training events at conferences in the field would facilitate increased training participation for scientists working in the area of fish heath management.

The majority of respondents clearly felt the need to improve their skills in diagnostic methods for bacterial and viral diseases, especially the newer molecular diagnostic techniques. A key issue that emerged from the survey was the stated desire of respondents to undertake training in epidemiology and risk analysis where this training is not currently available. This skill deficit has also been identified by the PANDA taskforce on epidemiology and risk analysis in aquatic animal diseases. Important facilitators of training included the availability of funding (especially in Southern European countries), the availability of more intensive workshops, and better information on training opportunities. Networking of experts and collaboration with industry to share knowledge were also identified as facilitators. Very few respondents considered that the availability of distance and e-learning would be of benefit to them in increasing their skills base.

It was also clear from the survey that respondents considered that the involvement of the EC would be positive in terms of both training policy and provision. In particular, a desire for harmonisation of methods, policies and regulations, training standards and qualifications across the European area was seen as important to improving the overall skills base and ultimately the level of fish health management and the quality and safety of fish and shellfish products. It was also clear from the survey that respondents saw EC involvement in policy on training and training provision as a means of securing a stable funding base for future training programmes.

Acknowledgements

I would like to acknowledge the financial support for this work provided through the Concerted Action Project PANDA SSPE-CT2003-50329. Many thanks to my fellow PANDA-ites for their help with the design and piloting of this survey, and their helpful input into the interpretation of the results.

Dr. Maura Hiney, National University of Ireland Galway, Galway City, Ireland
E-mail: maura.hiney@nuigalway

Dodet B, the OIE Scientific & Technical Department (eds): The OIE Global Conference on Aquatic Animal Health. Dev Biol (Basel). Basel, Karger, 2007, vol 129, pp 125-136.

Training Needs and Provision in Developing Countries of the Asia-Pacific Region

C. R. Lavilla-Pitogo

Fish Health Section, Aquaculture Department, Southeast Asian Fisheries Development Center (SEAFDEC), Tigbauan, Iloilo, Phillipines

Key words: fish health training, Asia-Pacific, e-learning, developing countries

Abstract: Training has played a significant role in the development of capacity in aquatic animal health in the Asia-Pacific region where most specialists have fisheries or a background in biology rather than in veterinary medicine. Training courses offered by various organizations, national institutes, universities and the private sector are aimed at providing graduates with skills in disease diagnostics using molecular methods, histopathology, epidemiology, immunology, as well as in disease prevention and control methods. Most training programmes either focus on diseases affecting specific commodities, such as shrimp, marine fish or molluscs, or on diagnostic methods for pathogens such as viruses. Because of the need to train a large pool of geographically dispersed participants, innovative and cost-effective ways of delivery like online and on-site training should be encouraged as well as workshops preceding or following meetings and symposia. One important aspect to be addressed is the translation of training materials to facilitate knowledge transfer to the farm level. Since the inadequate level of aquatic animal health expertise in the Asia-Pacific affects worldwide aquaculture, partnerships between governments, various international organizations and academia should be strengthened in order to fill the training gap.

Introduction

The Asia-Pacific region is responsible for more than 90% of world aquaculture production with a wide variety of species in different production systems. The fast-paced growth of aquaculture is plagued by previously unknown diseases due to inadequate biosecurity, sub-optimum environmental conditions and management, and widespread contamination of culture areas that share common waterways. Asian aquaculture has also been characterized by the emergence of transboundary diseases brought about by advances in live aquatic animal trade [1]. The major review on fish health management in the Asia-Pacific that was funded by the Asian Development Bank [2] recognized that diseases posed the biggest challenge for the growth of the aquaculture industry and that the ability of most governments to effectively overcome the disease and environmental problems was lacking. It was further recognized that training across a wide range of specialties in fish health needed to be implemented, with the significant involvement of personnel, in order to provide technical assistance to industry stakeholders. In the Asia-Pacific region where most specialists have backgrounds in fisheries or biology rather than in veterinary medicine, training has played a significant role in the development of capacity in aquatic animal health.

Major Training Providers

In 1985, the International Development Research Centre of Canada (IDRC) initiated the Asian Fish Health Network (AFHN) to promote high quality scientific research and the exchange of technical information among government and university scientists, diagnosticians, national policy makers and the members of the private sector. This programme led to significant progress in human capacity through degree programmes and training. At the Universiti Pertanian Malaysia (now Universiti Putra Malaysia) based at Selangor, Malaysia, a program was offered to develop post-graduate level staff from various countries in Asia with Masters and Doctorate degrees in Tropical Fish Health through fellowships from IDRC of Canada. Training under the IDRC programme included diagnostics for microbial, nutritional and environmental diseases. Histopathology was also an important area where capacity was advanced. Special training in biostatistics and experimental design was also introduced during a three week course at the University Sains Malaysia, in 1990.

The Aquatic Animal Health Research Institute (AAHRI) based at the Kasetsart University campus in Bangkok, Thailand, is the lead centre for disease research and diagnosis for the Department of Fisheries of Thailand. Through funding from the Food and Agriculture Organization (FAO), United Nations Development Programme (UNDP), Canadian International Development Agency (CIDA), IDRC of Canada, and later from the Overseas Development Administration (ODA) of the United Kingdom (presently known as the Department for International Development (DFID), in early 1992, AAHRI was established to become a centre of aquatic disease research for Southeast Asia. Aside from advancing knowledge and the understanding of new and existing infectious diseases in aquatic animals, developing effective disease control measures, and doing research to improve food quality and the safety of aquaculture products for domestic and export markets, AAHRI also provides an efficient fish disease diagnosis service to fish farmers and issues fish health and farm sanitary certificates to exporting farmers. Through its three groups composed of the fish health research group, the fish disease control and surveillance group and the drug and chemical control group, AAHRI offers workshops and training to local fish farmers and students. National and regional researchers from various countries are welcome to utilise the laboratory facilities, especially for research in

Epizootic Ulcerative Syndrome (EUS), for which AAHRI is the OIE reference laboratory. Training courses in shrimp health management are organised annually in collaboration with the Network of Aquaculture Centres in Asia-Pacific (NACA) and the University of Stirling. AAHRI also offers tailor-made aquatic animal disease training upon request.

AAHRI has published references that have become important resources for training such as *The Histology of Snakehead, A Manual of Hybrid Catfish Husbandry and Health, Histology of the Walking Catfish, Health Management in Shrimp Ponds, The Fish Disease Dictionary, Pathology and Histopathology of Epizootic Ulcerative Syndrome (EUS), the Technical Handbook of Diagnostic Procedures for Finfish Diseases,* and various disease manuals for farmers.

The Central Institute of Brackishwater Aquaculture (CIBA) under the Indian Council of Agricultural Research (ICAR) was established in 1987 to conduct research for development of brackish water aquaculture, to act as a repository of information on brackish water fishery resources with a systematic data base, and to undertake transfer of technology through training, education and extension education programmes. The Institute has ties and collaborates with other ICAR Fisheries Research Institutes as well as with international organizations such as the FAO-Bay of Bengal Programme, the NACA, the Government of France, AKVAFORSK of Norway and the World Bank. Aside from offering training programmes in brackish water aquaculture, CIBA also offers Aquatic Animal Health Management training as part of its extension services for State officials, faculty members and students of Fisheries Colleges and Agricultural Universities and also for farmers and entrepreneurs engaged in shellfish and finfish aquaculture activities.

The Department of Fishery Microbiology of the Karnataka Veterinary, Animal and Fisheries Sciences University is a United Nations Educational, Scientific, Cultural Organization (UNESCO) Microbial Resource Centre for Marine Biotechnology based in Mangalore, Karnataka, India that serves as an advanced centre for research and training. This UNESCO programme has conducted international training workshops for young researchers in Asia such as the Molecular Techniques in the Detection of Pathogens Associated with Seafood Workshop, in 1996; the Pathogens Associated with Seafood and Risk Assessment Workshop, in 1999; the Molecular Techniques in the Rapid Detection of Seafood Associated Pathogens, in 2001; the Water and Waste Water Microbiology Workshop, in 2003; and the Molecular Techniques in Aquaculture and Seafood Safety Workshop, in 2006.

Short-term training programmes are also offered for officers of various government departments, technicians from hatcheries and fish processing units, and scientists from universities and research institutions. Subjects offered include shrimp disease diagnosis using PCR and traditional methods, bacteriological techniques in aquaculture, molecular techniques for the rapid detection of pathogens associated with seafood, testing efficiency of probiotics and antimicrobial agents, microbiological and biochemical tests of water, and training in bioinformatics.

THE ACIAR MASTER CLASS ON EPIDEMIOLOGY IN TROPICAL AQUACULTURE

One of the major knowledge gaps among fish health workers in the Asia-Pacific region is epidemiology. The ODA Regional Seminar on EUS that was conducted in Bangkok in 1994 recommended that epidemiological expertise be developed in the region to support investigations of important fish diseases with complex etiologies, such as EUS. Furthermore, the FAO Regional Expert Consultation on Aquaculture Health Management in the Asia-Pacific [3] recognized the dearth of epidemiologists in aquatic animal health and recommended that efforts be made to rectify the situation. Thus, in July 1996, the Australian Centre for International Agricultural Research (ACIAR) organized and funded a master class aimed at senior aquatic animal health program managers, educators and researchers. ACIAR was then involved in key fish disease research in the region and within the ranks of its cooperating agencies in Australia were high level experts in veterinary epidemiology.

The master class was conducted at the AAHRI in Bangkok, Thailand, for two weeks and thirteen senior fish health specialists from the Asian region participated. The master class joined the AAHRI, the NACA and industry in a formal demonstration of the usefulness of epidemiology as a tool to better understand and solve major regional aquatic animal health problems. The workshop introduced participants to epidemiological theory and methods, and led to discussions on generic response strategies to fish disease epizootics and their management and containment at local, national and regional levels. This training event has spurred follow-up activities and ties with other regional and international organizations, and paved the way for a major shift in the perspective of disease analysis from focusing on the pathogen to emphasizing the fish and its relationship with its culture environment.

THE FISH HEALTH SECTION (FHS) OF THE ASIAN FISHERIES SOCIETY

One of the most significant activities of the FHS is the triennial Symposium on Diseases in Asian Aquaculture (DAA), six of which have been held so far, attended by recognized experts in various fields of fish health. In addition to providing a venue for the presentation of scientific papers and discussion of broad issues and specific topics related to fish health, it has also organised pre- and post-conference training sessions and workshops in order to maximize the value of travel time and expenses. At the fourth DAA in Cebu, the Philippines, in 1999, the first training program on Molluscan Health Management and the Risk Analysis Workshop organized by FAO were held. At the fifth DAA, in Gold Coast, Australia, in 2002, the FHS in collaboration with the organizers in Australia organized two satellite workshops: Epidemiology and Risk Assessment, and Phase II of the Asia-Pacific Regional Molluscan Health Management Training Program. In order to build a strong base of future researchers and trainers, the same group of participants attended Phases I and II of the training programme on Mollusc Health Management. Expertise on mollusc health management and pathology is generally wanting in Asia-Pacific.

At the sixth DAA Symposium, held in Colombo, Sri Lanka in 2005, a two-day pre-conference workshop on Fish Disease Diagnosis and Health Management was organized in collaboration with the Sri Lanka Ministry of Fisheries and the University of Kelaniya. Thirty-nine Sri Lankan participants participated in the workshop with international lecturers.

Training at the SEAFDEC Aquaculture Department

The Southeast Asian Fisheries Development Centre (SEAFDEC) is a regional treaty organization established in December 1967 to promote fisheries development in the region. The Member Countries are Brunei Darussalam, Cambodia, Indonesia, Japan, Lao PDR, Malaysia, Myanmar, the Philippines, Singapore, Thailand, and Vietnam. The Aquaculture Department in Iloilo, the Philippines was established in 1973 to conduct research, develop technologies, disseminate information, and train people in the farming of fishes, crustaceans, molluscs, and seaweeds for food, livelihood, equity, and sustainable development. Its mandates are to promote and undertake research on aquaculture relevant and appropriate to the region; encourage human resource development in aquaculture through training and extension; and disseminate and exchange information in aquaculture. To fulfill the mandate of developing human resources in aquaculture, the Government of Japan largely supported setting up training programs.

Traditional Fish Health Course

From 1987 to 2002, the Aquaculture Department of SEAFDEC offered 14 sessions of the Fish Health Management Training Course (FHMTC) at its main station in Iloilo, the Philippines. The course duration was from four to six weeks. The SEAFDEC worked closely with local, national and international organisations and invited lecturers to augment its pool of experts and to ensure the highest quality and relevance of its course content. The training program was designed to include 70% practical and 30% classroom type instruction covering topics on the various microbial pathogens and non-infectious disease agents, and their prevention and control. Field trips to grow-out farms and hatcheries were also part of the training. The curriculum was designed such that, at the end of the course, trainees were able to recognize diseased shrimp and fish, identify their causes, explain how the disease developed, and know the appropriate preventive and control measures to lessen the risk of these diseases. Emphasis was placed on sample preparation for submission to a laboratory for correct diagnosis. Aside from disease identification and control, relevant issues on health and the environment were added to the lectures to update the participants on new developments and trends.

For all its training courses, SEAFDEC awarded fellowships for participants from Member Countries through funds from the Government of Japan. Sixty-five percent of the total participants received these fellowships and their selection was based on the endorsement or nomination by representatives of Member Countries of the SEAFDEC Council. Other participants were funded by their own institutions and by national and international funding organizations. The number and distribution of participants in FHMTC are shown in Figure 1. In September, 1992, SEAFDEC conducted a workshop to assess the effectiveness of its training courses and to recommend ways to make training courses more responsive to the needs of the aquaculture industry. The workshop recognised the lack of skilled technicians in disease diagnosis [4] and the findings provided the basis for the continuation of training sessions in fish health at its headquarters in Iloilo, the Philippines. Through years of conducting FHMTC, the SEAFDEC has developed expertise in teaching and delivery. The collection of lecture notes and audio-visual aids has given rise to the book Health Management in Aquaculture [5] which has become an important reference for fisheries and veterinary students.

e-Learning

Shrinking fellowship and travel funds required a shift in training paradigm. Thus, the materials used in traditional FHMTC were transformed to produce AquaHealth Online (AHOL): a team developed and electronically delivered course on Health Management in Aquaculture. The course's pedagogy, modules, contents and delivery had already been presented elsewhere [6]. Among the many advantages of online course delivery is the elimination of travel and daily subsistence cost since the e-learners learn the modules and interact with specialists and mentors through the internet based discussion boards. More information about the course can be found at http://www.seafdec.org.ph/training/aquahealthonline.html. The general objective of transforming the course was to train a large pool of geographically dispersed participants at minimum cost. Figure 2 shows the distribution map of participants and their funding sources. Similar to FHMTC, funds were provided by the Government of Japan for fellowships of qualified participants from SEAFDEC Member Countries; however, 40% of participants came from the private sector and were funded by their respective organizations. One problem that became obvious with online course delivery was the lack of internet access and its prohibitive cost in some countries. Since there are no face-to-face meetings and all contact of students with the assigned mentors of each module was through an internet-based discussion board, failure of a participant to log-in results in non-participation and a lack of interaction. In the five completed sessions of AHOL, not one participant from Cambodia and Laos has passed the course (Fig. 3). E-learning, therefore, is not the way to reach those in countries with an under-developed web-based communication system. Furthermore, since all of the e-learners study while they are working, good time management is critical in order to cope with the additional load of reading modules, participating in the discussions, completing assigned tasks and accomplishing examinations.

Hands-on Training

The component of FHMTC that was obviously lacking in AquaHealth Online was hands-on activity, which comprised almost 70% of the traditional course. A workshop on Disease Control in Fish and Shrimp Aquaculture in Southeast Asia held in Iloilo City, the Philippines, in December, 2001, with 60 participants from 12 countries, strongly recommended the implementation of an international training course on the diagnosis of viral diseases. Thus, a two-week hands-on training curriculum was designed to develop capability in aquatic animal health diagnosis and management, especially for technical staff working at research centres and institutions in the Asian region and for participants who have passed AHOL. A total of 33 participants have attended the course since 2002 (Fig. 4).

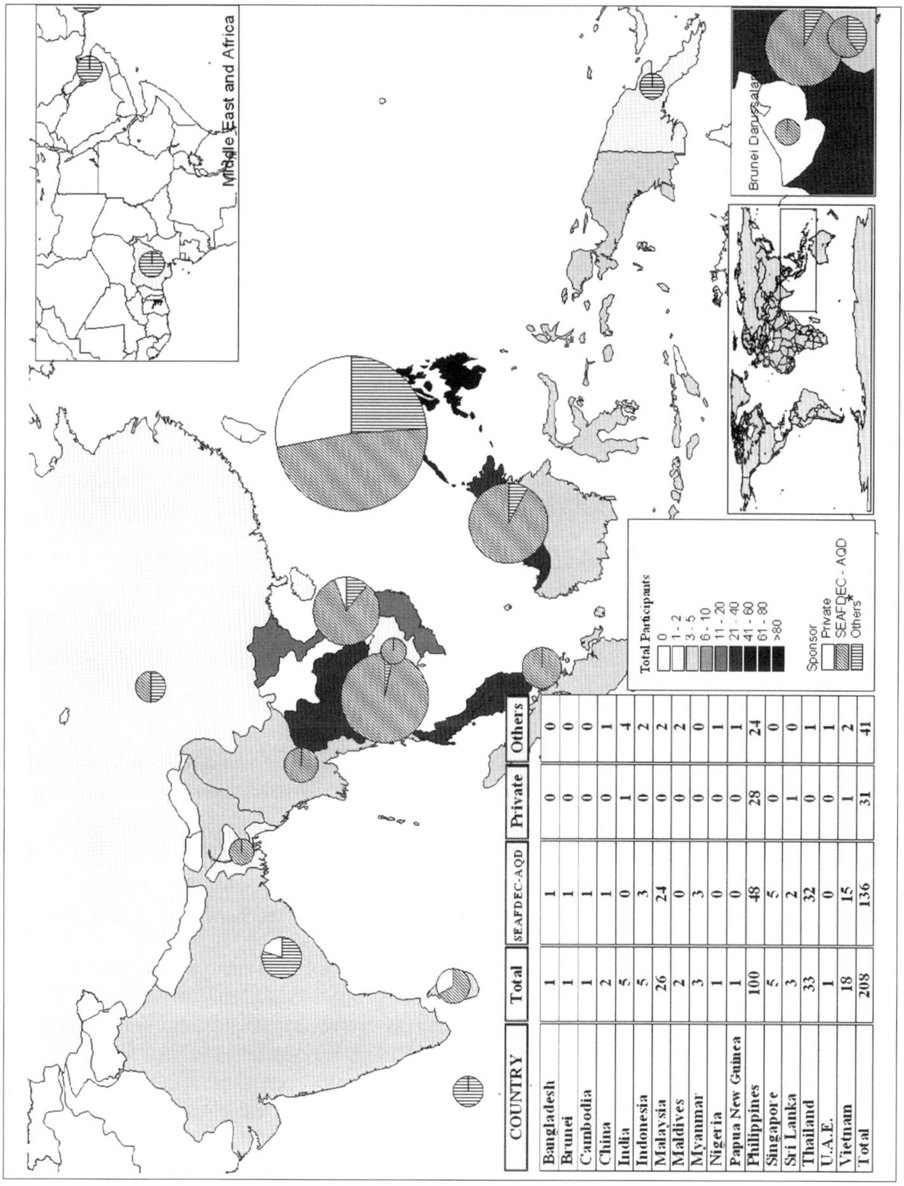

COUNTRY	Total	SEAFDEC-AQD	Private	Others
Bangladesh	1	1	0	0
Brunei	1	1	0	0
Cambodia	1	1	0	0
China	2	1	0	1
India	5	0	1	4
Indonesia	5	3	0	2
Malaysia	26	24	0	2
Maldives	2	0	0	2
Myanmar	3	3	0	0
Nigeria	1	0	0	1
Papua New Guinea	1	0	0	1
Philippines	100	48	28	24
Singapore	5	5	0	0
Sri Lanka	3	2	1	0
Thailand	33	32	0	1
U.A.E.	1	0	0	1
Vietnam	18	15	1	2
Total	208	136	31	41

Fig. 1: Distribution map of participants of the Traditional Fish Health Training Courses that were coducted by the SEAFDEC Aquaculture Department from 1987 to 2002.

On-site Training

In March, 2005, SEAFDEC launched the Human Resource Development for Sustainable Fisheries project in the Brunei-Indonesia-Malaysia-Philippines Economic Growth Area (BIMP-EAGA) with financial support from the ASEAN Foundation through the ASEAN-Japan Solidarity Fund. The on-site training sessions aimed at improving the capacity of front-line officers of various localities in the BIMP-EAGA to promote and assist aquaculture development. The thrust was to enhance the capability of government officers to advise farmers on good aquaculture practices to minimize the risk of disease and improve their farm's production. After the training session, the general consensus was that on-site training delivery was effective because of facilitated communication by translators. Because of this experience, SEAFDEC decided to embark on additional on-site training sessions in health management in Myanmar, Cambodia, Vietnam and the Lao People's Democratic Republic.

In addition to the organized training sessions, SEAFDEC also accepts internships and special on-the-job and on-demand training programmes for participants from the private sector and academia. For the past few years (2005-2007), SEAFDEC has conducted two-week enhancement training sessions for sixth-year veterinary students from the Aklan State University, Aklan, the Philippines, to introduce the students to aquaculture and the disease problems of this field, for which health care is comparatively insufficient compared with livestock and poultry.

Training Needs

Despite the various strategies that have been employed to develop manpower in aquatic animal health, there remains a need to advance larger efforts in training in the Asia-Pacific because growth of the industry has outpaced the availability of trained manpower to cope with the myriad of species being grown in different aquaculture systems. Up to now, most countries remain unable to cope with disease problems in aquaculture. Since many aquaculture techniques are easy to operate, aquaculture has become the source of livelihood for many poor people in rural communities. It is thus important, to train a pool of trainers who can deliver aquatic animal health services in the local language. Also, the existing manuals, field guides, and disease cards should be translated into local languages. An example of this is the monograph entitled Husbandry and Health Management of Grouper [7], a book that was written by experts from SEAFDEC commissioned by the Asia-Pacific Economic Cooperation (APEC). The book, originally written in English, has been translated to Pilipino, Thai, Chinese, Bahasa and Vietnamese. Translation of the book to Vietnamese was not part of the original publication package, but it was funded by the Ministry of Fisheries of Vietnam. This exemplifies that training and information resources can be further spread through government commitment and partnership.

Training for quarantine officers as well for staff who issue certification and conduct import risk analyses and zoning should be intensified now that several fast-growing, exotic species are available for the industry. Training activities, such as contingency planning and emergency preparedness, disease response and disease

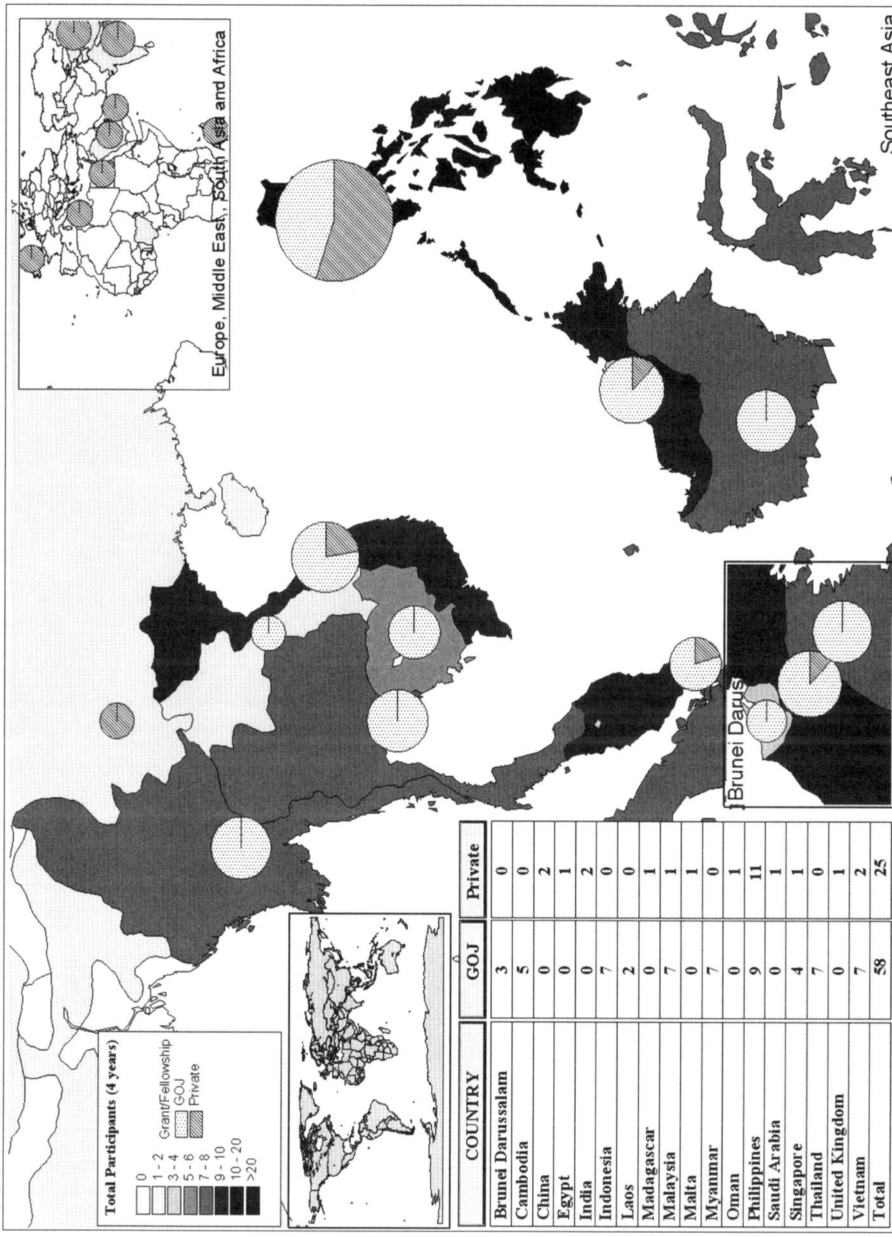

COUNTRY	GOJ	Private
Brunei Darussalam	3	0
Cambodia	5	0
China	0	2
Egypt	0	1
India	0	2
Indonesia	7	0
Laos	2	0
Madagascar	0	1
Malaysia	7	1
Malta	0	1
Myanmar	7	0
Oman	0	1
Philippines	9	11
Saudi Arabia	0	1
Singapore	4	1
Thailand	7	0
United Kingdom	0	1
Vietnam	7	2
Total	58	25

Fig. 2: Distribution map of participants of the AquaHealth Online course that were conducted by the SEAFDEC Aquaculture Department from 2002 to 2005.

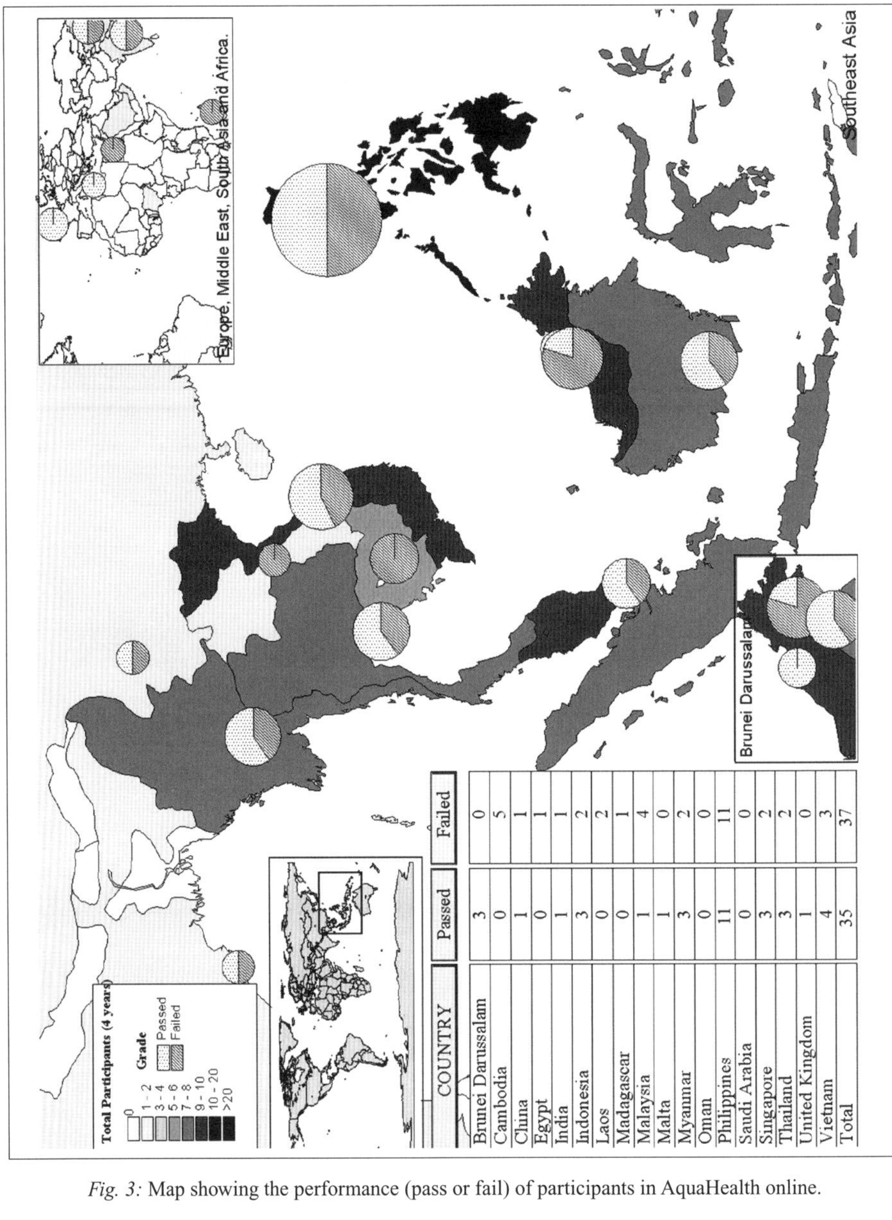

COUNTRY	Passed	Failed
Brunei Darussalam	3	0
Cambodia	0	5
China	1	1
Egypt	0	1
India	1	1
Indonesia	3	2
Laos	0	2
Madagascar	0	1
Malaysia	1	4
Malta	1	0
Myanmar	3	2
Oman	0	0
Philippines	11	11
Saudi Arabia	0	0
Singapore	3	2
Thailand	3	2
United Kingdom	1	0
Vietnam	4	3
Total	35	37

Fig. 3: Map showing the performance (pass or fail) of participants in AquaHealth online.

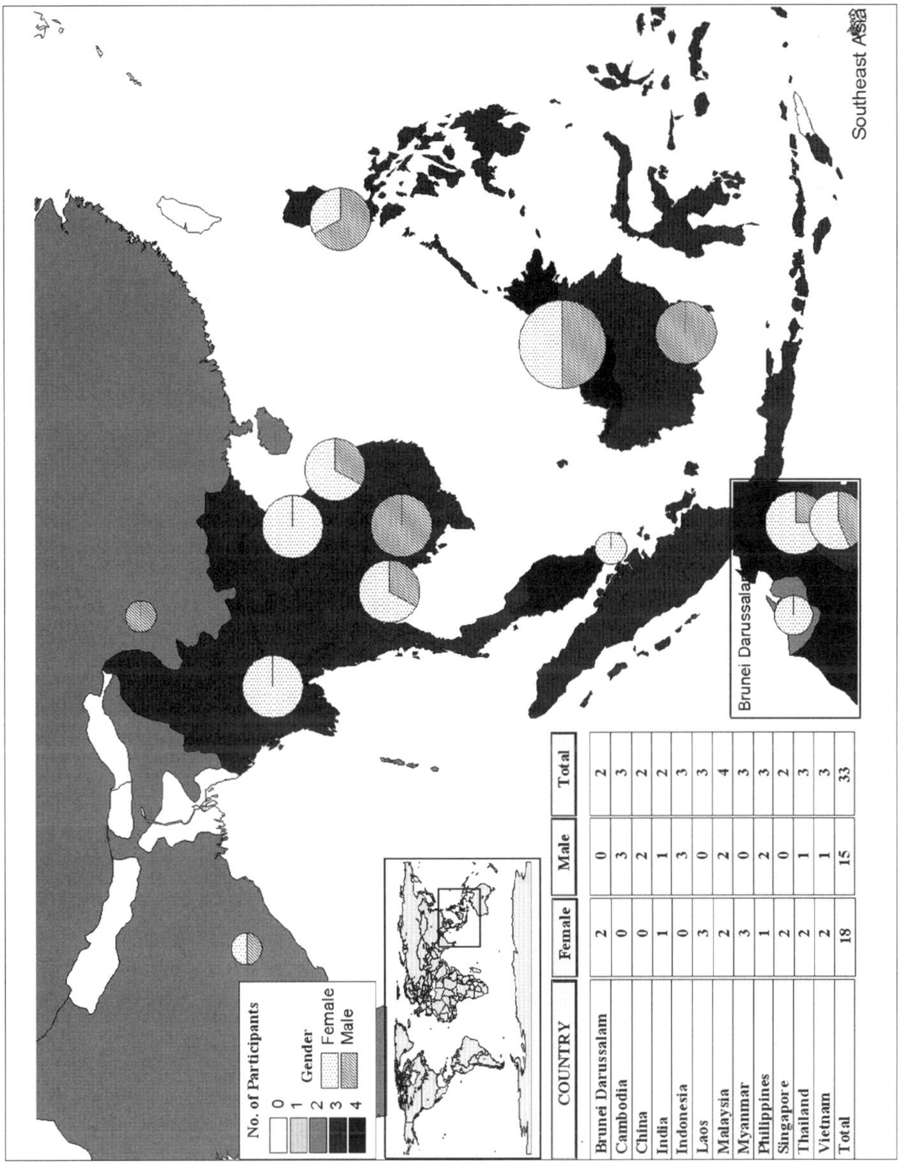

COUNTRY	Female	Male	Total
Brunei Darussalam	2	0	2
Cambodia	0	3	3
China	0	2	2
India	1	1	2
Indonesia	0	3	3
Laos	3	0	3
Malaysia	2	2	4
Myanmar	3	0	3
Philippines	1	2	3
Singapore	2	0	2
Thailand	2	1	3
Vietnam	2	1	3
Total	18	15	33

Fig. 4: Distribution map showing the participants in the Hands-on Training Session for Viral Diseases of Shrimp and Marine Fish

simulation exercises that are part of the routine capacity-building efforts of developed countries are yet to be introduced in most countries in the Asia-Pacific. The obvious dearth of aquatic animal health expertise in the Asia-Pacific, where most fish comes from, posses a problem to worldwide aquaculture; thus partnership of governments with various international organizations and the academia should be strengthened in order to fill the training gap.

Acknowledgement

The author thanks Joseph B. Biñas for preparing the GIS maps.

References

1 Subasinghe RP: Experiences in dealing with aquatic animal disease emergencies in Asia, in Subasinghe RP, Arthur JR (eds): Regional Workshop on Preparedness and Response to Aquatic Animal Health Emergencies in Asia. Food and Agriculture Organization, 2005, Fisheries Proceedings No 4, pp 67-72.

2 ADB/ NACA: Fish Health Management in Asia-Pacific: Report on a Regional Study and Workshop on Fish Disease and Fish Health Management. Network of Aquaculture Centres in Asia-Pacific, 1991, ADB Agriculture Department Report Series No. 1.

3 Tonguthai K: Training and Extension in Aquaculture Health Management in the Asia-Pacific: Present Status and Future Requirements, in Subasinghe RP, Arthur JR, Shariff M (eds): Health Management in Asian Aquaculture. Proceedings of the Regional Expert Consultation on Aquaculture Health Management in Asia and the Pacific. Food and Agriculture Organization, 1996, Fisheries Technical Paper No. 360.

4 Villegas CT, Castaños MT, Lacierda RB (eds): Proceedings of the Aquaculture Workshop for SEAFDEC/AQD Training Alumni. SEAFDEC Aquaculture Department, 1993.

5 Lio-Po GD, Lavilla CR, Cruz-Lacierda ER (eds): Health Management in Aquaculture. SEAFDEC Aquaculture Department, 2001.

6 Lavilla-Pitogo CR, Torres PL Jr: AquaHealth Online: A New Learning Environment for Capacity Building in Aquatic Animal Health, in Lavilla-Pitogo CR, Nagasawa K (eds): Transboundary Fish Diseases in Southeast Asia: Occurrence, Surveillance, Research and Training. SEAFDEC Aquaculture Department, 2004, pp 53-66.

7 APEC/SEAFDEC: Husbandry and Health Management of Grouper. APEC Singapore and SEAFDEC Aquaculture Department, 2001.

Dr. Celia R. Lavilla-Pitogo, Fish Health Section, SEAFDEC Aquaculture Department, Tigbauan 5021, Iloilo, Philippines
E-mail: celiap@aqd.seafdec.org.ph

Dodet B, the OIE Scientific & Technical Department (eds): The OIE Global Conference on Aquatic Animal Health. Dev Biol (Basel). Basel, Karger, 2007, vol 129, pp 137-146.

Opportunities for Training in Shrimp Diseases

D.V. Lightner, R.M. Redman

OIE Reference Laboratory for Shrimp Crustacean (Penaeid Shrimp) Diseases, Department of Veterinary Science & Microbiology, University of Arizona, Tucson, AZ, USA

Key words: shrimp diseases, training, penaeid shrimp, shrimp industry

Abstract : Opportunities for formal training in shrimp diseases were not available 30 years ago. This was because the shrimp farming industry was in its infancy with few significant disease issues and even fewer shrimp disease specialists investigating the causes of production losses. In 2006, more than two million metric tons of the marine penaeid shrimp were farmed, accounting for more than half of the world's supply. With most of the world's shrimp fisheries at maximum sustainable yields, the ratio of farmed to fished shrimp appears likely to continue to increase. The remarkable growth of sustainable shrimp farming was made possible through the development of methods to diagnose and manage disease in the world's shrimp farms. This occurred as the result of the development of training opportunities in shrimp disease diagnosis and control methods and the application of that knowledge, by an ever increasing number of shrimp diseases specialists, to disease management at shrimp farms. The first type of formal training to become generally available to the industry was in the form of special short courses and workshops. The first of these, which was open to international participants, was given at the University of Arizona in 1989. Since that first course several dozen more special short courses and workshops on shrimp diseases have been given by the University of Arizona. Dozens more special courses and workshops on shrimp diseases have been given by other groups, including other universities, industry cooperatives, governments and international aid agencies, in a wide range of countries (and languages) where shrimp farming constitutes an important industry. In parallel, graduate study programs leading to post graduate degrees, with shrimp disease as the research topic, have developed while formal courses in shrimp diseases have not become widely available in veterinary or fisheries college curricula in the USA and Europe, such courses are appearing in university programs located in some of the shrimp farming countries of SE Asia. The trend towards more formal training programs in shrimp diseases and disease management is likely to continue as the industry continues to mature and become increasingly sustainable.

INTRODUCTION

More than half of the world's production of penaeid shrimp now comes from farms. This is a noteworthy achievement for a major food producing industry that began only 35 years ago [1,2]. While the shrimp industry has experienced phenomenal growth, it has also been constrained by a number of infectious diseases. Paucity of knowledge on shrimp diseases, disease diagnosis, and disease prevention and control curtailed the industry's early development and contributed to the virus-caused pandemics that began in the late 1980s. These viral pandemics cost several billion dollars in lost revenue, millions of lost jobs, and even threatened the existence of some segments of the industry. The industry's ability to overcome the effects of the viral pandemics and subsequently grow in such a phenomenal manner is due to effective disease prevention and control [2,3]. The development of education and training programs that have produced an ever growing number of qualified shrimp disease diagnosticians and researchers has also contributed to this growth. These programs have largely been in the form of special workshops and short courses in shrimp pathology, disease diagnosis, and biosecurity. The first Shrimp Pathology Short Course was offered at the University of Arizona in 1989. Since that first Short Course, many more special short courses and workshops on various aspects of shrimp pathology, diagnostic methods and diseases management have been developed and given in many locations. Opportunities for advanced training in shrimp disease through this and numerous other short courses, workshops, and graduate programs now available globally, are contributing to an ever growing number of well qualified shrimp disease diagnosticians and researchers needed to support the continued growth and sustainability of shrimp aquaculture. Some of the major milestones in the history of the international shrimp farming industry and the nature and type of training opportunities available during those time periods are discussed in the present paper.

DISEASE ISSUES AND TRAINING OPPORTUNITIES IN THE FIRST 20 YEARS (1970 TO ~1985) OF SHRIMP FARMING: THE FIRST PERIOD

The commercial farming of penaeid shrimp began in the early 1970's. In the ensuing two decades, the industry experienced phenomenal growth. According to FAO statistics for 1985, in less than two decades the industry grew from its experimental beginnings to producing nearly 200,000 metric tons or ~25% of the world shrimp supply [1,4]. The dominant species cultured during the period of 1970 to ~1990 were the Giant Black Tiger Shrimp (*Penaeus monodon*), the Chinese White Shrimp (*Fenneropenaeus chinensis*), the Kuruma or Japanese Tiger Shrimp (*Marsupenaeus japonicus*), the Pacific White Shrimp (*Litopenaeus vannamei*) and the Pacific Blue Shrimp (*L. stylirostris*). Virtually all of the main shrimp producing countries in Asia and the Americas relied exclusively on locally sourced wild shrimp for the seed stock (usually postlarvae or "PLs") used to stock farms. In Asia, PLs were typically produced in hatcheries from wild or captive-wild mated adult broodstock, while in the Americas, much of the industry relied on PLs which were collected directly from shrimp nursery grounds in coastal areas and estuaries prior to being used to stock shrimp farms, or on PLs produced from captive-wild broodstock in hatcheries or "laboratories." Grow-out technologies were relatively simple. In Asia, semi-intensive or intensive culture methods, generally in small ponds, were the typical types of grow-out systems employed, while in the Americas large semi-intensive ponds were the most typical culture system [2,4,5].

During these years there were significant disease events caused by several major pathogens in Asia and the Americas [6-9]. The principal diseases had a wide range of etiologies, including viral, bacterial, fungal, parasitic, epicommensal, and nutritional agents (Table 1). Among the virus diseases, Monodon baculovirus (MBV), baculoviral mid-gut necrosis virus (BMNV), and hepatopancreatic parvo-like virus (HPV) in Asia, baculovirus penaei (BP) and hematopoietic necrosis virus (IHHNV) in the Americas were the principal virus-caused diseases, while the main bacterial diseases were caused by several species of bacteria in the genus *Vibrio*. Diseases caused by fungi, especially larval mycosis in hatcheries, posed a major constraint to shrimp culture until methods for its prevention and control were developed in the mid 1980's. By 1990, highly efficacious methods for the prevention of larval mycosis were adopted by the industry, and the disease is now only rarely encountered [7,10,11].

Table 1: Major shrimp diseases in Asia & the Americas during the industry's first period (1970 - ~1985).

Asian Diseases		**Western Hemisphere Diseases**	
Viral	**Other Diseases**	**Viral**	**Other Diseases**
MBV	Vibriosis (*Vibrio* spp.)	BP	Vibriosis (*Vibrio* spp.)
BMNV	Larval mycosis	IHHNV	Larval mycosis
	(Sirlopidium sp.)		*(Lagenidium callinectes)*
HPV	Fusariosis		Fusariosis
	(Fusarium solani)		*(Fusarium solani)*
	Surface epicommensal & fouling organisms		Surface epicommensal & fouling organisms

Virus caused diseases were especially significant. Baculoviral diseases due to MBV, BMNV (in Asia) and BP (in the Americas) caused significant losses, especially in the larval and early PL stages. Improved culture practices were developed during this period in which improved sanitation of spawned eggs, nauplii and culture systems were employed, along with the detection and destruction of infected broodstock and/or spawns [2,6,12]. IHHNV was particularly significant in the Americas where it caused catastrophic losses in most locations where *L. stylirostris* was farmed. Despite the generally superior size and ease of *L. stylirostris* culture, its far greater susceptibility to IHHN disease was the principal reason why *L. vannamei*, with it relatively greater resistance to IHHN disease, became the dominant penaeid species reared in the Americas by the early 1980's [2,5,7,13].

Vibrio spp. were the predominant cause of bacterial disease, and they were responsible for significant losses in all phases of shrimp culture. In hatcheries, vibriosis was commonly managed by the routine use of a variety of antibacterial compounds administered directly to the larval rearing tank water. At the farm level in both Asia and the Americas, vibriosis emerged as a significant disease during this period. The use of medicated feeds containing antibacterial compounds like oxytetracycline, chloramphenicol, and various nitrofurans and sulfa drugs, were adopted as a routine management tool for vibriosis [7,10].

During this period, disease had adverse effects on the development of the industry, especially in the last few years with the viral pandemics [6-10,13]. Shrimp diseases were of relatively minor importance for most of the industry and there were very few shrimp disease experts or diagnostic laboratories available, and even fewer opportunities for training in shrimp disease. There were a few graduate programs in which students could perform research on the diseases of shrimp that were emerging as major problems in the budding shrimp disease industry. Most of these programs were located at universities in the USA, France, Taiwan, and Mexico.

The Role of Education and Training in Shrimp Diseases in Shaping the Future of the Shrimp Farming Industry during the Second Period (~1985 to Present)

The series of viral pandemics that began around 1986 forever changed the way that shrimp were farmed (Table 2). In 1986 Taiwan had become the dominant producer of farmed shrimp in the world with production levels approaching 100,000 metric tons per year. However, in 1986 a severe viral pandemic caused the collapse of the industry. MBV was implicated by Taiwanese scientists and government authorities as the cause of the epizootic [6,7,14], but because MBV has never been shown to cause catastrophic disease in *P. monodon*, it seems more likely that some other viral disease similar to Yellow Head Disease (YHD), which emerged a few years later as a major disease in SE Asia, was the actual cause of the collapse [6-9,11].

In 1991, YHD emerged as a major disease in *P. monodon* farms in Thailand. The next year White Spot Disease (WSD) appeared in East Asia and its viral agent, WSSV (White Spot Syndrome Virus) quickly spread across East and Southeast Asia causing a pandemic over the next four to six years that resulted in multibillion dollar losses in production and export revenues to the shrimp farming industries of the affected countries [2,6-8,11].

The same year (1991) that YHV emerged in SE Asia, Taura Syndrome Disease (TS, caused by Taura syndrome virus, TSV) appeared in Ecuador. By 1992, TS had spread to a number of farms in the Taura River region and it was recognized as a major new disease of *L. vannamei*. By 1994, TS had spread to most of the shrimp farming regions of the Americas causing nearly $1 billion in lost production [5,13,15,16]. During the same year the etiology of TS was shown to be a virus. Litigation by Ecuadorian shrimp farmers against several producers and users of fungicides used on banana plantations near the first affected farms in Ecuador began and fuelled a heated controversy that clouded the understanding of the etiology of TS for the next eight years [5].

Table 2: The viral pandemics of the first and second periods of shrimp farming (~1985 to present).

Virus	Year Disease Appeared	Region	Estimated Production Loss Since Year of Emergence
IHHNV	1981	Americas	$500 million to 1 billion
MBV & unknown agent	1986	Taiwan	$800 million
YHV	1991	Thailand, SE Asia	$500 million
TSV	1991/92	Americas	$1-2 billion
TSV	1999	Taiwan, E & SE Asia	$>1billion
WSSV	1992/93	E, SE & Central Asia	$12 billion
WSSV	1999	Americas	$2-3 billion
IMNV	2002	Brazil	$>100 million

In 1995, the first case of WSD was diagnosed in the Americas, but it was not until early 1999 that WSSV reached the major shrimp farming regions [17,18]. Within a year WSSV had devastated the hemisphere's major shrimp farming countries. In less than two years, WSSV caused an additional $1-2 billion in lost production and the loss of at least 500,000 jobs [5,19]. By January, 2005, WSD had reached Brazil, the last major shrimp producing country in the Americas. Dr. Grace Lo (author of the OIE Manual chapter on White Spot Disease) estimated that by 2006 WSD had caused cumulative losses of $12 billion to the shrimp farming industries of Asia and the Americas [12].

Several other important diseases emerged during this period. Necrotizing hepatopancreatitis (NHP) was first recognized as a distinct disease in 1985 in *L. vannamei* cultured in Texas. By 1995, NHP was shown to be caused by an intracellular, rickettsial-like alpha proteobacterium and to occur in many of the shrimp farming regions of the Americas located in semiarid regions or in areas with an extended hot, dry season [5,7,10].

In 2002, another major viral disease, Infectious Myonecrosis (IMN caused by IMNV), emerged in shrimp farms in north-central Brazil [5,20]. Within two to three years, IMN had spread eastward into at least five Brazilian states in the northeast of the country and accounted for approximately 20,000 metric tons, or about $40 million, in lost production [21]. By 2006, losses due to IMN in Brazil were estimated to exceed $100 million (ABCC, Brazil, unpublished). That same year, IMNV, and the disease it causes, was reported from Indonesia, reportedly having been introduced there with illegally imported *L. vannamei* broodstock from Brazil [22].

Challenges and Disease Management Following the Viral Pandemics; the Current Period

The viral pandemics collectively caused nearly $15 billion in economic losses to shrimp producing countries and the loss of a half a million to a million jobs [3,5,6,8,9,12]. Because of the economic significance of the viral pandemics and their potential for further spread, the diseases caused by IHHNV, TSV, WSSV, YHV, MBV and BP have become listed by the World Animal Health Organisation (OIE). Reflecting the importance of the penaeid shrimp aquaculture industry, eight of the nine OIE listed crustacean diseases are diseases of penaeid shrimp (Table 3) [23].

Table 3: OIE Listed (or Proposed for Listing) Crustacean Diseases as of December 2006 [21].

Disease Name	Agent / Type	Principal Host(s)
Taura Syndrome	TSV / Dicistroviridae	*Litopenaeus vannamei* & *L. stylirostris*
White Spot Syndrome/ Disease	WSSV / Nimaviridae	All penaeids & most decapods
Spherical Baculovirosis	MBV / Baculoviridae	*Penaeus monodon*
Tetrahedral Baculovirosis	BP/ Baculoviridae	American penaeids
Yellow Head Disease	YHV/GAV / Roniviridae	*P. monodon*
Infectious Hypodermal & Hematopoietic Necrosis	IHHNV / Parvoviridae	*L. vannamei, L. stylirostris* & *P. monodon*
Necrotizing Hepatopancreatitis*	NHP-B / Alpha-Proteobacterium	All penaeids
Infectious Myonecrosis*	IMNV / Totiviridae	*L. vannamei* & *L. stylirostris*
Crayfish Plague	Aphanomyces astaci / phycomycetous fungus	European crayfish

* Under study for possible listing by OIE.

In the wake of the extraordinary losses that occurred as a result of the viral pandemics, the industry began to mature, becoming much more sustainable and technology-based. The industry has largely recovered from the major viral pandemics and it now produces nearly two million metric tons per year, twice what it produced in 2002 and nearly two-thirds of the world's total shrimp supply [1,4]. The adoption of new shrimp farming technologies and the abandonment of practices which posed high disease risks has contributed to the industry's recovery and current expansion. Among the most notable changes in culture practices has been the shift of the industry away from using wild stocks for seed production to the use of domesticated stocks [2,4,5]. This has been a consequence of the ever increasing incidence of diseases like WSSV and IHHNV in wild shrimp stocks, which has made the collection of wild PLs and adult broodstock for the production of PLs for use as seed stock a risky practice. With the declining dependence of the industry on wild stocks in Asia and in the Americas, the use of domesticated lines of specific pathogen-free (SPF) *L. vannamei* recently surpassed *P. monodon* as the dominant farmed shrimp species in Asia [4]. This paradigm switch in the species being farmed occurred within five years after the SPF *L. vannamei* stocks were introduced in quantity to Asia. The use of SPF *L. vannamei* has led to improved predictable crops in virtually all areas that were once dominated by the culture of *Fe. chinensis* and *P. monodon*. The term "biosecurity" was not used in shrimp farming a decade ago, but today most farms incorporate some form of the practice for disease exclusion and management [2, 3].

The Development of Training Opportunities

The University of Arizona (UAZ) began to offer short courses for the training of research scientists and diagnosticians in shrimp pathology in the most recently developed and appropriate diagnostic procedures, in biosecurity, and in disease prevention and control methods for the major diseases of cultured penaeid shrimp. These courses have been made available to scientists and staff of domestic and foreign governments, and to the domestic and foreign shrimp culture industries. The first UAZ Shrimp Pathology Short Course was given in 1989. Since then, UAZ has taught 18 of its regular Shrimp Pathology Short Courses on the University of Arizona campus and an additional 26 short courses and special workshops on shrimp pathology and shrimp disease diagnostic methods. To date UAZ has trained around 475 graduates from 53 countries or territories in its regular Short Course. With students from UAZ special workshops and short courses given abroad, that makes around 1,030 students, government officials, and shrimp farm and diagnostic lab personnel who have received formal training in shrimp pathology and diagnostic methods from UAZ.

Other Training Programs

Since 1990, other universities, governments, international aid organizations (such as FAO), several large shrimp farming companies, and companies that make and sell diagnostic kits or instruments (i.e. PCR thermocyclers) for shrimp diseases have offered shrimp pathology short courses and special topic workshops. Some examples of the best known shrimp pathology short courses and workshops are listed in Table 4. The number of trainees (students, government officials, diagnosticians, etc.) that have received formal training in shrimp diseases, diagnosis and management is estimated to be in the tens of thousands with more being added each year.

Table 4: Examples of some shrimp pathology short courses and workshops.

Course	Location
Shrimp Pathology Short Course	University of Arizona, Tucson, AZ, USA
Biology and Pathobiology of the Penaeid Shrimp	Mahidol University, Bangkok, Thailand
Shrimp Health Management & Disease Diagnostics	Harbor Branch Oceanographic Institution, Fort Pierce, FL, USA
Annual Texas Shrimp Farming Short Course	University of Texas, Port Aransas, TX, USA
Shrimp Health Management Training Workshop	NACA, Bangkok, Thailand
FAO sponsored workshops	Honduras, Nicaragua
Special Training in Shrimp Diseases	SEAFDC, Philippines

Post graduate programs at universities in numerous countries have offered advanced degrees on topics that include shrimp diseases. Countries with universities with graduate programs that have produced significant numbers of graduates include: the USA, France, England, Scotland, the Netherlands, Mexico, Ecuador, Colombia, Taiwan, China, Korea, Japan, Australia, Thailand, India, French Polynesia, and Indonesia. Much of the current scientific literature reflects the importance of university research in advancing the knowledge base in shrimp disease and in producing the personnel needed for future research and development.

Veterinarians have entered the field of shrimp pathology and their numbers are increasing, especially in developing nations. Many of the more important diagnostic laboratories and many government agencies that oversee shrimp farming employ veterinarians. The field of shrimp pathology is expanding as rapidly as the global shrimp farming industry and consequently there are likely to be many opportunities for veterinarians for careers in the field. Ironically, few veterinary schools (at least in the USA and Europe) recognize this opportunity and offer courses and/or specialization in aquatic animal diseases.

Training in Shrimp Diseases and Industry Development - Future Visions

The current trends in shrimp farming and shrimp disease control are likely to continue well past 2010. By that time, most if not all, farmed shrimp will be from domesticated, genetically improved lines that are SPF for most significant shrimp diseases. The most significant shrimp diseases will be managed by exclusion. Diagnostic methods for most major diseases will be further developed and refined;

highly sensitive methods will be commonplace in central diagnostic laboratories; and simple, relatively sensitive methods will be in routine use in shrimp hatcheries and farms for the rapid diagnosis of significant disease threats. For non-excludable diseases, more and better probiotic products will be available, as will a number of "vaccines" that will effectively prevent infection by some disease agents. Antibiotic use in shrimp farming will likely be reduced in culture systems where probiotics and "vaccines" can be effectively used. However, when they are used, antibiotics will be better controlled to minimize environmental concerns (i.e. development of resistant bacteria) and to insure that antibiotic residues are below tolerance levels set by importing countries.

Culture systems will become more intensive, using less land, less water, and less feed for each ton of shrimp produced. Biosecurity for the purpose of disease prevention will be routine on all shrimp farms. Such biosecure, intensive to super-intensive culture systems will produce shrimp efficiently and at low cost so that shrimp may come to compete head-to head with other high protein meat products like beef, swine, poultry and salmon. Disease will continue to cause losses to the shrimp farming industry. The recent emergence of a number of new diseases such as infectious myonecrosis (IMN), Spiroplasmosis, Monodon slow growth syndrome, etc., and the development of new strains of "old" diseases like TSV remind us that the job of disease management and control will be an ongoing task for as long as shrimp are farmed. The need for personnel that are well trained in shrimp diseases (i.e. researchers, diagnosticians, regulatory officials, and on-farm biologists) will continue to increase with the growth of the shrimp farming industry and these personnel will be instrumental in ensuring the industry's sustainability.

Acknowledgements

Grant support for this review was provided by the United States Marine Shrimp Farming Consortium under Grant No. 2004-38808-02142 from the Cooperative State Research, Education and Extension Service, US Department of Agriculture.

References

1 Tacon AGJ: Aquaculture production trends analysis, in Review of the State of World Aquaculture: FAO Fisheries Circular No. 886, Rev. 2, Rome, 2003, pp 5-29.

2 Lightner DV: Biosecurity in shrimp farming: pathogen exclusion through use of SPF stock and routine surveillance. J World Aquaculture Soc 2005; 36:229-248.

3 Lee CS, O'Bryen PJ (eds): Biosecurity in Aquaculture Production Systems: Exclusion of Pathogens and Other Undesirables. The World Aquaculture Society, Baton Rouge, 2003.

4 FAO: State of world aquaculture. FAO Fisheries Technical Paper 500, Food and Agriculture Organization of the United Nations, Rome, 2006.

5 Lightner DV: The penaeid shrimp viral pandemics due to IHHNV, WSSV, TSV and YHV: history in the Americas and current status, in: Sakai Y, McVey JP, Jang D, McVey E, Caesar M (eds): Proceedings of the Thirty-second US Japan Symposium on Aquaculture. US-Japan Cooperative Program in Natural Resources (UJNR), U.S. Department of Commerce, NOAA, Silver Spring, 2003; pp 6-24, and at: http://www.lib.noaa.gov/japan/aquaculture/aquaculture_panel.htm

6 Flegel TW: Detection of major penaeid shrimp viruses in Asia, a historical perspective with emphasis on Thailand. Aquaculture 2006; 258:1-33.

7 Lightner DV (ed): A Handbook of Shrimp Pathology and Diagnostic Procedures for Diseases of Cultured Penaeid Shrimp. World Aquaculture Society, Baton Rouge, 1996.

8 Flegel TW: Major viral diseases of the black tiger prawn (*Penaeus monodon*) in Thailand. World J Microbiol Biotechnol 1997;13:433-442.

9 Flegel TW, Alday-Sanz V: The crisis in Asian shrimp aquaculture: current status and future needs. J Appl Ichthyol 1998;14:269-273.

10 Brock JA, Lightner DV: Diseases of crustacea. Diseases caused by microorganisms: Diseases of Marine Animals, Vol. III, Kinne O(ed). Biologische Anstalt Helgoland, Hamburg, 1999; pp 245-349.

11 Bondad-Reantaso MG, McGladdery SE, East I, Subasinghe RP (eds): Asia Diagnostic Guide to Aquatic Animal Diseases. FAO Fisheries Technical Paper 402, Supplement 2. Rome, FAO, 2001.

12 OIE (Office International des Epizooties): Manual of diagnostic tests for Aquatic Animal diseases, 5th edition. Office International des Epizooties, Paris, 2006.

13 Lightner DV, Redman RM: Shrimp diseases and current diagnostic methods. Aquaculture 1998;164:201-220.

14 Chen SN, Chang PS, Kou GH, Lightner DV: Studies on virogenesis and cytopathology of *Penaeus monodon* baculovirus (MBV) in the Giant Tiger Prawn (*Penaeus monodon*) and the Red Tail Prawn (*Penaeus penicillatus*). Fish Pathol 1989;24:89-100.

15 Hasson KW, Lightner DV, Mohney LL, Redman RM, Poulos BT, Mari J, Bonami JR: The geographic distribution of Taura Syndrome Virus (TSV) in the Americas: determination by histology and *in situ* hybridization using TSV-specific cDNA probes. Aquaculture 1999;171:13–26.

16 Lightner DV: The penaeid shrimp viruses TSV, IHHNV, WSSV, and YHV: current status in the Americas, available diagnostic methods and management strategies. J Appl Aquaculture 1999;9:27-52.

17 GAA (Global Aquaculture Alliance): Shrimp white spot virus confirmed in Central America. GAA Newsletter, 1999, vol. 2 issue 2.

18 GAA (Global Aquaculture Alliance): Shrimp white spot disease in Latin America an update. GAA Newsletter, 1999, vol. 2 issue 3.

19 Vidal OM, Granja CB, Aranguren F, Brock JA, Salazar M: A profound effect of hyperthermia on survival of *Litopenaeus vannamei* juveniles infected with White spot syndrome virus. J World Aquacult Soc 2001;32: 364-372.

20 Poulos BT, Tang KFJ, Pantoja CR, Bonami JR, Lightner DV: Purification and characterization of infectious myonecrosis virus of penaeid shrimp. J Gen Virol 2006;87:987-996.

21 Nunes A J P, Cunha-Martins P, Vasconselos-Gesteira TC: Carcinicultura ameacada. Rev Panoram Aquic 2004; 83:37–51 (in Portuguese).

22 Saengchan S, Phewsaiya K, Briggs M, Flegel TW: Outbreaks of infectious myonecrosis virus (IMNV) in Indonesia confirmed by genome sequencing and use of an alternative RT-PCR detection method. Aquaculture (2007; in press).

23 OIE (Office International des Epizooties): Aquatic Animal Health Code, 9th edition. Office International des Epizooties, Paris, 2006.

Dr. Don. V. Lightner, OIE Reference Laboratory for Shrimp Crustacean (Penaeid Shrimp) Diseases, Department of Veterinary Science & Microbiology, University of Arizona, Tucson, AZ 85721 USA
E-mail: dvl@u.arizona.edu

Dodet B, the OIE Scientific & Technical Department (eds): The OIE Global Conference on Aquatic Animal Health. Dev Biol (Basel). Basel, Karger, 2007, vol 129, p 147.

Session VI

Aquatic Animal Welfare

Chairperson: *D. Lightner*, USA

Dodet B, the OIE Scientific & Technical Department (eds): The OIE Global Conference on Aquatic Animal Healths. Dev Biol (Basel). Basel, Karger, 2007, vol 129, pp 149-161.

OIE Involvement in Aquatic Animal Welfare: The Need for Development of Guidelines Based on Welfare for Farming, Transport and Slaughter Purposes in Aquatic Animals

T. Håstein

National Veterinary Institute, Oslo, Norway

Key words: aquatic animal welfare, OIE, guidelines, standards

Abstract: Globally there has been increasing agreement that aquatic animals are entitled to certain welfare considerations and standards. This trend will most likely grow stronger in the years to come. The World Animal Health Organisation (OIE) has realised that animal welfare issues are receiving increased public attention by governments as well as non-governmental and consumer organisations. Animal welfare was identified as a priority in the 2001-2005 OIE Strategic Plan. OIE Member Countries decided that the OIE must provide international leadership on animal welfare. Animal protection includes important scientific, ethical, economic and political dimensions and thus a need to establish guidelines in the field of welfare. The OIE established a permanent Working Group on Animal Welfare (2002) to coordinate and manage animal welfare activities. It was indicated that the welfare of animals used in agriculture and aquaculture should be prioritized and that the development of policies and guiding principles on transportation, humane slaughter and killing for disease control purposes was a primary task. Thus, the OIE established two *ad hoc* Groups to draft the guiding principles on the humane slaughter of fish for human consumption, killing fish for disease control purposes, and land and sea transport based on the generic OIE guiding principles and policies for animal welfare.Below, the scope and development of these Guidelines, the OIE guiding principles for the welfare of aquatic animals as well as the OIE *in house* procedures for the approval of a set of guidelines to be incorporated into the *OIE Aquatic Animal Health Code* will be described in more detail.

Introduction

Over the past few years, there has been increasing global agreement that aquatic animals are also entitled to certain welfare considerations and standards, a trend that will be growing stronger and stronger in the years to come. This has inevitably led to a rationale for the development and adoption of aquatic animal welfare guidelines both nationally and internationally.

Involvement of Governmental Bodies in Animal Welfare

Certain countries have already included aquatic animals in their animal protection acts, such as Australian Capital Territory and Queensland, New Zealand, Norway and the United Kingdom (UK). The Animal Health and Welfare Act 2006 of Scotland, also applying in England and Wales, states the following:

> *"The Act makes it an offence to cause or permit any unnecessary suffering to a protected animal. The Act defines a protected animal as a vertebrate animal other than man, which is commonly domesticated in the British Islands or under the control of man or not living in a wild state. The definition includes all farmed fish."*

The Norwegian Animal Welfare Act (1974) that included fish as well as decapods states that the main principle and the scope of the Act according to Article 2 are as follows: *"Animals shall be treated well, and consideration shall be given to the instinctive behaviour and natural needs of animals, so that there is no risk of causing them unnecessary suffering."*

In the European Union (EU), the 1997 Treaty of Amsterdam states that *"Member States shall pay full regard to the welfare of animals..."* [1].

OIE Involvement in Animal Welfare

The World Organisation for Animal Health (OIE) realised that animal welfare issues were under increased public attention. Thus, the OIE identified in its 2001-2005 Strategic Plan [2] that animal welfare was a priority task; the OIE, as the international reference organisation for animal health and zoonotic diseases, had to provide international leadership on animal welfare. Even though animal welfare is not covered by the WTO SPS Agreement, the OIE Member Countries wished to have guidelines and recommendations to assist them in bilateral negotiations.

It was recognised that the OIE needed to develop a detailed vision and strategy incorporating and balancing these dimensions and to establish guidelines in the field of welfare as animal protection is a complex, multi-faceted public policy issue which includes important scientific, ethical, economic and political dimensions. The OIE thus established a permanent Working Group on Animal Welfare (AWWG) in 2002 to coordinate and manage the animal welfare activities of the OIE.

Since the OIE International Committee had indicated that the welfare of animals used in agriculture and aquaculture should be prioritized and that the topics of transportation, humane slaughter and killing for disease control purposes were to be addressed first, followed by housing and management, the AWWG recognised development of policies and guiding principles as primary tasks. On the basis of this, the AWWG established a work programme for 2003 describing how the prioritized topics should be addressed by means of *ad hoc* Groups with experts on welfare issues within the prioritized areas. The recommendations of the AWWG were adopted at the 71st OIE General Session in May, 2003, at which a member representing welfare interests of aquatic animals was elected to the AWWG.

The terms of reference given for the work of the *ad hoc* Groups for terrestrial animals on introduction to welfare, transport and slaughter for consumption/ killing included fish, as resources permitted or when the expertise was available, but it was soon clear that separate *ad hoc* Groups for aquatic animals were needed.

Development of the OIE Guidelines on Aquatic Animal Welfare

In February 2004, a decision was made to establish *ad hoc* Groups to prepare an introduction to OIE guidelines for the welfare of aquatic animals; guidelines on the transport (air, land, and sea) of fish; guidelines on the slaughter of fish for consumption and killing fish for disposal; and guidelines on aquatic animal production. So far no *ad hoc* Group has been established on fish production. The *ad hoc* Groups on the transport and slaughter/killing of fish were established in March, 2005, and had their first and only meeting in June, 2005. The *ad hoc* Groups prepared draft guidelines based on similar guidelines already prepared for terrestrial animals. The drafts were presented to the Aquatic Animal Health Standards Commission (AAHSC) at their meeting in August, 2005, but were not addressed in detail. At the September meeting of the AWWG, the drafts were then discussed and amended. The amended versions were again presented to the AAHSC in March, 2006, but it was not until their meeting in October, 2006, that the Commission discussed the drafts on the basis of comments from the OIE Member Countries [3].

Since the AAHSC agreed with the comments received from the OIE Member Countries, the drafts will go back to the AWWG which will further address the issues raised and provide scientific justification for the comments. This process will be carried out over 2007, so final drafts will not be adopted until May, 2008, at the earliest.

Main Points in the Process of Drafting the Guidelines

The terms of reference for drafting the guidelines are as follows: create a first output, a draft of guiding principles rather than a prescriptive approach to limits, specifically addressing the humane slaughter/killing and transport of fish for human consumption based on the generic OIE guiding principles and policies for animal welfare; focus on the commercial large scale slaughter/killing and transport of fish; create a final output, a draft of standards/guidelines for the *Aquatic Animal Health*

Code based on approved guiding principles; identify future directions in which the *ad hoc* Groups might need to move; and produce drafts for review by the OIE Working Group and then by the OIE Aquatic Animal Health Standards Commission.

The large scale slaughter for consumption of cold water fish species (i.e., salmonids) and warm water fish species (bass, bream, carp, etc.) will be covered. As resources permit, and when expertise is available, harvesting procedures for crustaceans (shrimp, lobster and crabs) will be addressed.

The OIE Welfare Guiding Principles

The draft of OIE guiding principles states that there is a relationship between aquatic animal health and aquatic animal welfare and that the international five freedoms in principle also apply to aquatic animals. The draft further states that the internationally recognized "three Rs" (Refinement; Reduction; Replacement) provide valuable guidance for the use of aquatic animals in science and that the scientific assessment of aquatic animal welfare involves diverse elements to be considered. There is no doubt that the use of aquatic animals contributes to the well-being of people and that improvements in aquatic animal welfare will improve productivity, food safety, etc., and lead to economic benefit.

The scientific basis for the draft guidelines states that welfare is a broad term describing how well aquatic animals will cope with their environment, management and handling and that the welfare of such animals can be scientifically evaluated with regard to aquaculture, research, harvest, and recreational fisheries to establish standards. The health status of aquatic animals is an indicator of their welfare. Although heavily disputed [4], recent publications using primarily neuroanatomy, neurophysiology and behaviour, [1,6] indicate that finfish may be sentient. Research is still required on the ability of aquatic animals to feel pain and to be sentient, but nevertheless studies have shown that they fulfil criteria for nociception and thus have a potential for the perception of pain. When performance indicators and measurements of optimal welfare are in place, they can be applied for the evaluation of practices in aquaculture, research and recreational fisheries.

Proposed Guidelines for the Slaughter of Fish for Human Consumption and Killing Fish for Disposal

As in terrestrial animal production, aquatic animals are purposefully killed for two primary reasons: for human consumption or to control/eradicate devastating diseases in both wild and farmed populations. The guiding principle for optimal slaughter is to avoid unnecessary stress and pain in connection with the slaughtering process; sedation should render instantaneous unconsciousness lasting until death [7]. A method that only gradually results in unconsciousness may be allowed, if the method in itself does not result in stress or pain [8].

For the guidelines, it is necessary to have a set of definitions; these will be placed with the other definitions in the *Code* if and when the guidelines are approved. *Article 1* gives a general description of the principles for slaughter that apply to finfish species slaughtered in slaughterhouses during the pre-slaughter, slaughter and transport processes; all processes must be done without undue stress. Furthermore, it is emphasised that personnel involved must be experienced and competent in the transport and handling of fish and familiar with the OIE guidelines and applicable legislation. *Article 2* covers the transport of fish for slaughter, which should be in accordance with the transport guidelines. In order to carry out the humane slaughter of fish it is important that the design of the holding facilities are as appropriate as possible prior to slaughter and hold the maximum number of fish in relation to the throughput of the slaughterhouse without compromising the welfare of the fish. *Article 3* describes in some detail important factors regarding the design of nets and holding tanks, water quality, sensory stimulation (lighting and noise) and systems for moving fish including pumps and pipes. *Article 4* describes procedures for unloading and moving of fish into the slaughterhouse. It is necessary that such processes should minimise fish health and welfare outcomes due to crowding and handling. This means that fish should be allowed to swim into the stunning device, if possible, to avoid unnecessary handling stress. *Article 5* gives a summary of acceptable stunning methods for fish and their respective welfare issues (Table 1). A key fish welfare requirement is that the personnel carrying out the stunning methods are competent for their job.

Table 1: A summary of acceptable methods for stunning fish and their respective welfare issues

Stunning method	Fish welfare concerns/implications	Applicable species
Percussive stunning	Hand operated equipment may be hampered by uncontrolled movement of the fish. Unconsciousness may not be achieved due to too weak a blow to the head. Injuries may occur.	Salmonids Halibut
Spiking (Iki-Jime)	Inaccurate application may cause injuries. May be hampered by uncontrolled movement of the fish. Difficult to apply.	Salmonids Tuna
Electrical stunning	Difficult to control and apply correctly in the field. Optimal control parameters unknown. May be hazardous to operating personnel.	Salmonids
Free bullet	Shooting distance and calibre are a concern. Noise of guns may cause stress reaction. May be hazardous for operating personnel.	Tuna

In *Article 6* a reference is made to the draft Guidelines for the humane killing of fish for disease control purposes. However, some general considerations regarding the appropriateness and effectiveness of equipment (use, maintenance, etc.), signs of correct stunning (opercular activity and visual evoke response (VER), loss of vestibulo-ocular reflex (VOR, eye rolling), and loss of tail reflex are given with regard to mechanical stunning, percussive stunning and spiking, coring, and Iki-Jime. Here, it is important to stress that bleeding should only be performed on fish that have been effectively stunned. Figures 1 and 2 show the principles for percussive stunning and spiking of Atlantic salmon and tuna, respectively. In addition to the different types of stunning methods, methods other than stunning have been used for the sedation of fish prior to slaughter. A summary of such methods is established in *Article 7* (Table 2). Not all methods used for the immobilisation of fish prior to slaughter are deemed acceptable from a welfare point of view and in *Article 8* several methods, procedures and practises considered unacceptable on fish welfare grounds due to aversive effects, are listed (use of CO2, live chilling/CO2, asphyxiation, exsanguination, etc.). The use of CO2 in Norway will thus be abandoned when slaughtering fish from 2008.

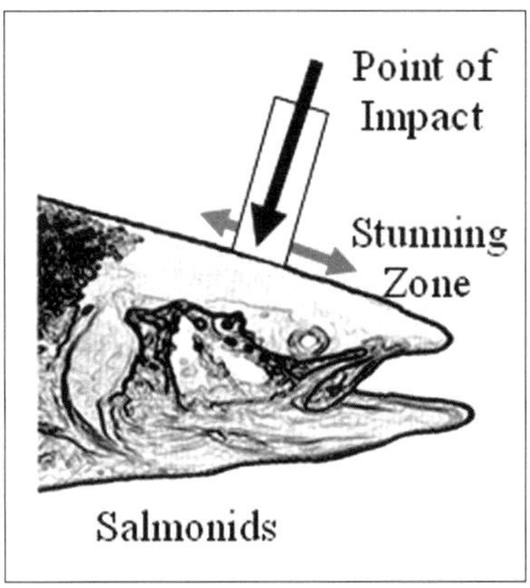

Fig. 1: The principle of percussive stunning of Atlantic salmon

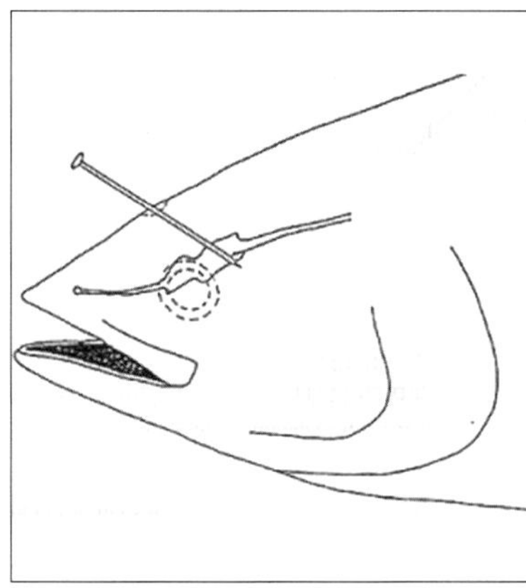

Fig. 2: The principle of spiking of tuna

OIE Draft Guidelines on Killing Fish for Disposal

Even when it is important to control a disease that is exotic or of socio-economic importance due to mortality, infectivity or lack of treatment, the organised killing of affected fish should be carried out on the basis of welfare criteria. The methods to be used are, in principle, the same as those accepted for slaughter for human consumption. However, for biosecurity reasons, diseased fish should be killed first, followed by the rest of the fish in due order. In order to prevent the spread of disease to the environment or other neighbouring aquaculture establishments,killing for control purposes should preferably take place on-site and measures should be taken to ensure that infected animals are collected and treated in an optimal way to prevent further spread of disease/disease agents.

Table 2: A summary of methods other than stunning used for the sedation, anaesthesia or immobilisation of fish.

Method	Application/effect	Fish welfare concerns/ implications	Key fish welfare requirements	Applicable species
Live chilling	Recoverable immobilisation prior to stunning/ slaughter.	Fish have not lost sensation. Season and species dependent.	Competent personnel and suitable control equipment/process	Salmonids/ cod/wolff-ish/ halibut
Aqui-S	Recoverable sedation/anaesthesia prior to stunning/ slaughter.	Fish may recover sensation prior to slaughter.	Control of dose. Competent personnel	Most fish species
CO2	Recoverable immobilisation prior to stunning/ slaughter.	Adverse effects. Fish become exhausted and die due to hypoxia and suffocation. Fish may not lose sensation	Competent personnel	Most fish species
Combination of CO2/O2 - Live chilling	Recoverable immobilisation prior to stunning/ slaughter	Adverse effects. Fish may not lose sensation. Season and species dependant.	Competent personnel	Salmonids
Electrical harpoon	Irrecoverable electrocution applied to the head prior to slaughter.	Good accuracy required to ensure fish killed	Competent personnel	Large tuna

As in the draft guidelines on slaughter, the draft guidelines on killing fish for disposal have a set of definitions that will be placed with the other definitions in the *Code* if and when the guidelines are approved. *Article 1* covers the general principles of the humane killing of finfish for disease control purposes and includes the need and content of contingency plans, disease strategies that include welfare issues, competencies of personnel involved, operational procedures including how killing should be carried out (quickly, immediate death) and proper carcass handling. Although the mass killing of fish may not distress the public as when such operations are carried out on terrestrial animals, the procedures should be done with as little public attention as possible. *Article 2* and *Article 3* give an overview over the responsibility of the *Competent Authority Official* regarding the activities on the premises that should be in accordance with OIE welfare and bio-security guidelines and the responsibility and competence of the operational team and aquatic animal technicians (team leader, veterinarians/fish health biologists, aquatic animal technicians, personnel responsible for the killing, and carcass disposal personnel), respectively. *Article 4* covers the operational guidelines including planning the killing and how to kill single fish versus the mass killing of fish. While single fish can be killed by a blow to the head, the mass killing of fish depends on the farming system and chemicals/equipment needed for the killing,

Table 3: A summary of acceptable killing methods for fish*

Species	Method	Animal welfare concerns/ implications	Additional comments
Salmonids, cod (gadids) and flatfish	Anaesthetic overdose using benzocaine, metacaine, iso-eugenol.	Considered to have a low impact on welfare but mode of operation of chemicals in all species is not known.	Applicable to all sizes of fish
	Percussive stunning.	Should be properly applied to be humane and effective. Low impact on welfare.	Suitable for fish handled individually
	Electrical stunning.	The equipment should be maintained and applied correctly to produce an effective stun and kill. Low impact on welfare. Suitable in salt water.	May be hazardous to personnel. Applicable to all sizes
Tuna	Spiking, coring, Iki-Jime.	When applied properly, the fish are killed instantly.	Applicable to all sizes
	Free bullet.	When applied properly, the fish are killed instantly.	Applicable to all sizes. Operator safety needs to be addressed.
Cyprinids	Anaesthetic overdose using benzocaine, metacaine, iso-eugenol.	Considered to have a low impact on welfare but mode of operation of chemicals in all species not known.	Applicable to all sizes
Eels	Decapitation.	Negative impact on welfare. Acceptable if preceded by anaesthesia.	
	Electrical stunning.	Eels are resistant to electrical stunning and require high currents for at least five minutes to achieve insensibility. Negative impact on welfare.	May be hazardous to personnel.
	Percussive stunning.	Low impact on welfare.	Suitable for fish handled individually.
Ornamentals	Anaesthetic overdose using benzocaine, metacaine, iso-eugenol.	Considered a low impact on welfare but mode of operation of chemicals in all species not known.	Applicable to all sizes.

* The order of description of the methods is not in an order of acceptability from a fish welfare point of view

Appendix VII (contd)

Species	Method	Animal welfare concerns/implications	Additional comments
Other species	Spiking, coring and Iki-Jime (tuna).	When applied properly, the fish are killed instantly.	
	Percussive stunning.	Should be properly applied to be humane and effective. Low impact on welfare.	Suitable for fish handled individually
	Electrical stunning.	The equipment should be maintained and applied correctly to produce an effective stun and kill. Low impact on welfare.	May be hazardous to personnel. Applicable to all sizes.
	Anaesthetic overdose using benzocaine, metacaine,	Considered to have a low impact on welfare but mode of operation of chemicals in all species not known.	Applicable to all sizes
	iso-eugenol.		
Newly hatched fry/eggs of any fish species	Maceration.	Low impact on welfare.	

Note: The table does not represent an exclusive list of acceptable methods

and the species and number of fish to be killed. As mentioned previously it is also necessary to register the absence of respiratory movement, visual evoked response, vestibulo-ocular reflex and tail reflex and muscular movements. The *Articles 5-9* describe different stunning methods that may be used for the mass killing of fish as well as unacceptable methods (*Article 8*). The methods may either be mechanical stunning methods, (percussive stunning, spiking, coring, Iki-Jime, and free bullet), electrical stunning or chemical methods. Article 10 gives a summary of acceptable methods for the mass killing of fish (Table 3). It is important that fish killed for biosecurity reasons be adequately handled; Article 11 refers to the OIE Guidelines for the handling and disposal of carcasses and waste of aquatic animals under preparation. Fig. 3 shows a model for the disposal of carcasses by burial.

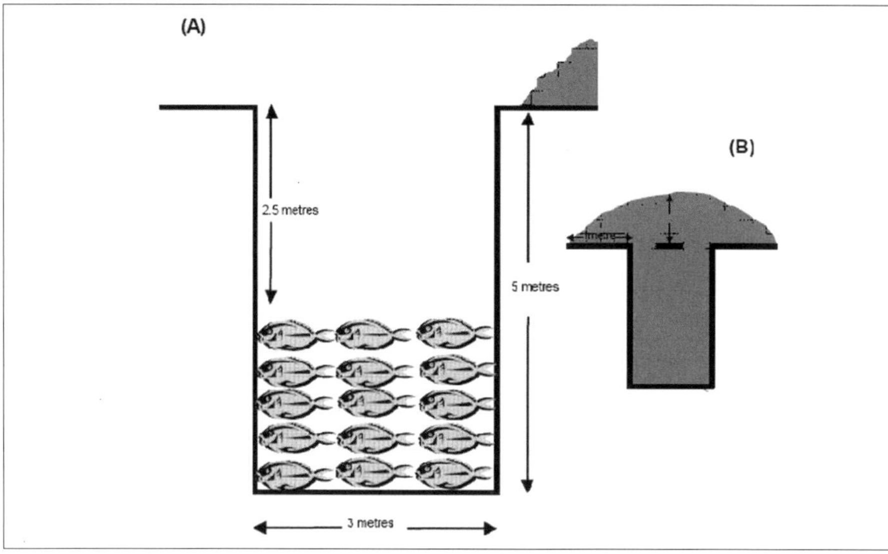

Fig. 3: Model of pit for disposal of carcasses by burial: (A) open pit; (B) freshly closed pit (Source: Aquavetplan 2002)

The OIE Draft Guidelines for the Land Transport of Fish

The OIE Draft Guidelines for the Land Transport of Fish were first intended to apply to salmonids and cyprinids but they may also apply to other fish species. The land transport guidelines also start with a set of important definitions, followed by comments on the distance of transport (Article 1), while *Articles 2-3* cover the responsibilities prior to, during and after transport as well as training and practical experiences needed (by owners, managers, aquatic animal technicians, transport companies, vehicle owners/drivers, and Competent Authorities).

In order to optimally transport live fish, appropriate planning is required regarding the type of vehicle, the route and duration of transport, emergency procedures and plans to identify adverse events. Vehicle design and maintenance (appropriate to the species), water quality factors, equipment on the vehicle/container and necessary documentation are also important, and all mentioned factors above are included in *Article 4*.

Articles 5-8 cover routines for the loading and unloading of fish including crowding, equipment, water quality, fish density during transport, and loading procedures as well as post journey activities including health checks of the fish prior to departure, during and after the journey, monitoring of water quality criteria and emergency procedures. The emergency procedures include notification of the Competent Authority, killing procedures to be used under such circumstances and notification to the place of arrival. In order to have appropriate documentation on health status, records should be kept and recommendations for handling fish showing clinical signs of disease are proposed as well as the needs for cleaning and disinfection.

Since any act of transport may go wrong and cause a dispute, procedures for action to be taken in the event of an inability to unload a consignment are laid down in *Article 9*. Such disputes should be settled by using the OIE dispute settlement mechanisms if international travel is involved.

The OIE Draft Guidelines for the Transport of Fish by Boat

The drafted guidelines for the transport of fish by boat are in principle the same as those laid down above for land transport.

Future OIE Guidelines to be Prepared

In the future, there may be a need for guidelines for the air transport of ornamentals as well as guidelines on crustaceans, specifically covering the transport of live crustaceans, the handling and killing of live lobsters for human consumption and killing for disposal.

Before guidelines concerning welfare issues for live crustaceans are established, the question of whether such guidelines are necessary will be raised. From the author's point of view, welfare is an integral part of crustacean health and the development of a set of guidelines will represent a precautionary principle of unacceptable handling and treatment of crustaceans. There is no doubt that crustaceans have a nervous system and a nociceptive system (capacity to detect and respond to noxious or adverse stimuli) and that they possess the features of a neurochemical system involved in pain perception. Thus they may feel pain. Demands from international bodies (i.e. the EU and the UK), as well as the fact that consumers are increasingly concerned by welfare aspects linked to food production, may lend momentum to the development of such guidelines even though it is not currently a priority for the OIE.

Future guidelines should cover important definitions; farmed and wild crustaceans; moving and handling of crustaceans prior to killing; requirements for live crustaceans transported in containers; methods for keeping live crustaceans prior to processing; and general principles for the humane killing of crustaceans (single individuals, mass killing) including a description of killing methods and documentation regarding welfare issues in the event of inadequate killing.

Requirements for the effective use of methods for the mass killing of live crustaceans should be given. For the time being chemical and electrical stunning/killing methods are the ones that should be considered, from a welfare point of view. Chemical killing methods may not be suitable for killing crustaceans bound for human consumption and thus electrical stunning/killing may be a method of choice as such equipment is now available on the market. For killing individuals, mechanical methods as shown in Fig. 4 may be used. Although dropping decapods (lobsters, crabs, shrimps) into boiling water has been the most common method of killing for human consumption, this method is not considered as appropriate as it is questioned whether they feel pain when boiled. It is still not known whether the vigorous whipping of the tail seen in lobsters upon boiling is a result of pain or a stress reaction is still not known. The method may be acceptable for small crustaceans, however. Thus, the boiling of large crustaceans unless sedated (i.e. by ice slurry), the sectioning of crabs before the nerve centres have been destroyed, the transverse sectioning of lobsters and crayfish and serving live crustaceans at the table are not acceptable from a welfare prospective.

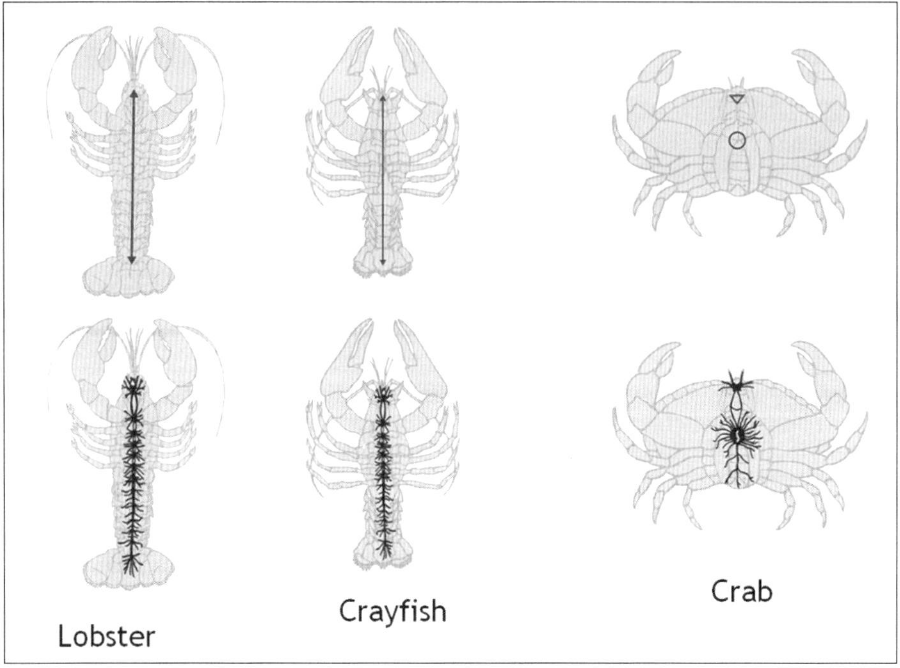

Fig. 4: Species specific mechanical methods for killing of single individuals, destruction of nerve centres in crayfish, crab and lobster. Upper row shows points of destruction (Upper line) and lower road shows the nerve centres in the mid-line (Lower line).

CONCLUSION

In conclusion, a set of international guidelines for aquatic animals reflecting welfare issues are needed because aquatic animals have their own value beyond the economic value for human beings; aquatic animals are entitled to moral respect and welfare considerations; ethical principles ensuring the health and welfare of fish, including their humane slaughter should govern the aquaculture industry despite historical, cultural and regulatory differences between countries. In order to be accepted by the international community, such standards must be based on science.

ACKNOWLEDGMENTS

I would like to thank Dr. Eva-Maria Bernoth, Australia, for use of the figure from Aquaplan 2002, Drs Lauritz Sømme & Heidi Sjursen for use of the drawings of the crustacean nerve system and Dr. Ida Skaar for preparation of the drawings of crab, crayfish and lobster.

References

1 Treaty of Amsterdam amending the Treaty on European Union, the Treaties establishing the European Communities and certain related acts. Protocol annexed to the Treaty of the European Community. Protocol on protection and welfare of animals. Official Journal C 340, 10/11/1997 pp 0110.

2 Håstein T, Scarfe AD, Lund VL (in press): Science-based assessment of welfare: Aquatic animals. Rev Sci Tech 2005;24(2).

3 Rose JD: The neurobehavioral nature of fishes and the question of awareness and pain. Rev Fisheries Sci 2002;10 (1):1-38.

4 OIE Strategic Plan 2001-2005. Please have the author complete/check this reference and verify the location of it in the text.

5 Chandroo KP, Duncan IJH, Moccia RD: Can fish suffer? Perspectives on sentience, pain, fear and stress. Appl Anim Behav Sci 2004;86:225-250.

6 Report of the Meeting of the OIE Aquatic Animal Health Standards Commission, Paris, 2-6 October 2006. Please complete reference.

7 Sømme LS. Sentience and pain in invertebrates: Report to Norwegian Scientific Committee for Food Safety, Norwegian University of Life Sciences, Norway, 2005.

8 Garseth ÅH: New sedation methods allowed in fish [in Norwegian]. Norsk Vet. Tidskr. 2003;8:586-588.

9 Van de Vis JW, Kestin S, Robb D, Oehlenschläger J, Lambooij B et al: Is humane slaughter of fish possible for industry? Aquacult Res 2003;34 (3):211-220.

Pr. Tore Håstein, National Veterinary Institute, PO box 8156 DEP, N-0033 Oslo, Norway
E-mail: tore.hastein@vetinst.no

Dodet B, the OIE Scientific & Technical Department (eds): The OIE Global Conference on Aquatic Animal Health. Dev Biol (Basel). Basel, Karger, 2007, vol 129, pp 163-170.

The OIE's Involvement in Aquatic Animal Health

E.-M. Bernoth

President, OIE Aquatic Animal Health Standards Commission, c/o Office of the Chief Veterinary Officer, Australian Government Department of Agriculture, Fisheries and Forestry, Canberra, Australia

Key words: OIE, aquatic animal health, Aquatic Code, Aquatic Manual

Abstract: The OIE develops normative documents relating to rules that Member Countries can use to protect themselves from diseases without setting up unjustified sanitary barriers. For aquatic animal disease, the *Aquatic Animal Health Code* and the *Manual of Diagnostic Tests for Aquatic Animals* are prepared by the Aquatic Animals Commission, with the assistance of internationally renowned experts, the OIE's other Specialist Commissions, and in consultation with OIE Member Countries. These standards are described in detail. There are currently 27 OIE Reference Laboratories and one Collaborating Centre for aquatic animal diseases, providing a network of expertise in aquatic animal health. The OIE is committed to raising awareness about aquatic animal health and assisting Member Countries to fulfill their international obligations. Members of the Aquatic Animals Commission regularly present on the activities of the Aquatic Animals Commission at the Conferences of the OIE Regional Commissions and at scientific venues. Regional initiatives conducted in concert with other organisations complement the OIE's involvement in aquatic animal health. A range of interesting challenges lies ahead.

Background

The World Organisation for Animal Health (OIE) is an intergovernmental organisation, created in 1924, of currently 169 Member Countries. Its main objectives are to ensure transparency in the global animal disease situation; to collect, analyse and disseminate veterinary scientific information; to provide expertise and encourage international solidarity in the control of animal diseases; within its mandate under the World Trade Organization's Agreement on the Application of Sanitary and Phytosanitary Measures (WTO SPS Agreement), to safeguard world trade by publishing health standards for international trade in animals and animal products; to improve the legal framework and resources of national Veterinary Services; to provide a better guarantee for the safety of food of animal origin; and to promote animal welfare through a science-based approach.

The International Committee is the highest authority of the OIE. It comprises the Delegates of all OIE Member Countries. The General Session of the OIE International Committee lasts five days and is held every year in May, in Paris. Voting by Delegates within the OIE International Committee respects the democratic principle of "*one country, one vote*". However, most decisions are made by the OIE International Committee on the basis of consensus, avoiding the need for the casting of votes by its Delegates.

Among the functions of the OIE International Committee is the election of the members of the OIE's four Specialist Commissions. The role of these Specialist Commissions is to use current scientific information to study problems of epidemiology and the prevention and control of animal diseases, to develop and revise the OIE's international standards, and to address scientific and technical issues raised by Member Countries.

The Fish Diseases Commission was established as an OIE Specialist Commission in 1960 because of the increasing awareness of the importance of international trade in fish. In 1988, the scope of the Commission was extended to include diseases of molluscs and crustaceans, and in 2003 the Commission was renamed as the Aquatic Animal Health Standards Commission (in brief, the Aquatic Animals Commission). Qualifications of the Commission's Members, its Terms of Reference and Internal Rules are published on the Commission's pages on the OIE website (http://www.oie.int/aac/eng/en_fdc.htm).

The OIE's Aquatic Standards

The OIE develops normative documents relating to rules that OIE Member Countries can use to protect themselves from diseases. By applying these rules, OIE Member Countries can be assured that their measures do not represent unjustified sanitary barriers, because the OIE normative documents are recognised as "international standards" under the agreements of the WTO. The aquatic standards (the *Aquatic Animal Health Code*, in brief, the *Aquatic Code*) and the *Manual of Diagnostic Tests for Aquatic Animals* (in brief, the *Aquatic Manual*) are prepared by the Aquatic Animals Commission with the assistance of internationally renowned experts, individually, or through *ad hoc* groups. The views of OIE Member Countries are systematically sought through the circulation of draft and revised texts to OIE Member Countries' Delegates. Delegates are expected to then circulate those drafts to relevant experts in their country for comment and consolidate comments into their country's response back to the OIE. The standards are finally adopted by the OIE International Committee at the annual General Assembly of all Delegates of OIE Member Countries. The value of the OIE standards is therefore twofold: the measures published in the OIE standards are the result of consensus among the veterinary authorities of OIE Member Countries; and the OIE standards constitute a reference within the WTO SPS Agreement as international standards for animal health and zoonoses.

The OIE *Aquatic Animal Health Code*

The aim of the *Aquatic Code* is to assure the sanitary safety of international trade in aquatic animals (fish, molluscs and crustaceans) and their products. This is achieved through the detailing of health measures to be used by the veterinary or other competent authorities of importing and exporting countries so that the transfer of agents pathogenic for animals or humans is minimised, while unjustified sanitary barriers are avoided. The *Aquatic Code* makes reference only to the aquatic animal health situation in the exporting country, assuming that either the disease is not present in the importing country or is the subject of a control or eradication programme. Therefore, when determining its import measures, an importing country should do so in a way that is consistent with the principle of national treatment and the other provisions of the SPS Agreement. The *Aquatic Code* is updated regularly, and a new edition is published each year, both in hard copy and on-line [1].

Part 1 of the *Aquatic Code* contains general provisions for aquatic animal health, while Part 2 details recommendations applicable to specific diseases. Appendices on blood sampling and vaccination and on inactivation of pathogens are contained in Part 3, and Part 4 provides model international aquatic animal health certificates.

Part 1 of the Aquatic Code

Section 1.1 of Part 1 of the *Aquatic Code* provides contextual definitions of the terms or expressions used. Section 1.2 describes "Notification systems", commencing with the statement that "*Countries shall make available to other countries, through the OIE, whatever information is necessary to minimise the spread of aquatic animal diseases and their aetiological agents and to assist in achieving better world-wide control of these diseases.*" This important "ground rule" is followed by detailed reporting requirements for OIE Member Countries. These rules specify the events in which immediate notification (within 24 hours) of the OIE is required. The overall purpose of these provisions is transparency about the animal health situation worldwide. While the necessity for such transparency is particularly obvious in clinical outbreaks of disease, this section of the *Aquatic Code* points out that the presence of an infectious agent, even in the absence of clinical disease, should also be reported. Section 1.2 then presents the disease listing criteria and the diseases listed by the OIE.

Section 1.3 presents "Obligations and ethics in international trade", which includes information on certification procedures. The aquatic animal health situation in the exporting country, in the transit country or countries and in the importing country should be considered before determining the requirements that have to be met for trade. This Chapter then continues with "Responsibilities of the importing country", for example, that the import requirements included in the international aquatic animal health certificate should assure that commodities introduced into the importing country comply with the national level of protection, and that importing countries should restrict their requirements to those justified for such a level of protection. If these are stricter than the OIE standards, guidelines and recommendations, then they should be based on an import risk analysis. Also detailed are the "Responsibilities of the exporting country", notably that it is prepared to supply certain information to importing countries on request. Responsibilities in the case of an incident occurring after importation are also laid down. The second Chapter in Section 1.3 specifies certification procedures.

Section 1.4 describes the principles of conducting risk analyses and provides detailed guidelines for each step, i.e. hazard analysis, risk assessment, risk management and risk communication. Two further Chapters in this section provide guidance on the evaluation of competent authorities and on zoning.

Section 1.5 is about "Import/export procedures" and describes aquatic animal health measures applicable before departure, during transit, and on arrival. Some of these are very detailed and technical requirements; for example, disinfection of transporters, treatment of transportation water, and discharge of infected water (Chapter 1.5.1), while others are more general requirements to be met before and at departure (Chapter 1.5.2), for example, that each country should only authorise the exportation of live aquatic animals and aquatic animal products that are correctly identified, and inspected according to the procedures outlined in the *Aquatic Code* and *Aquatic Manual*. Chapter 1.5.5 describes aquatic animal health measures applicable on arrival, for example, that an importing country should only accept into its territory, live aquatic animals that have been subjected to examination by a member of the personnel of the Competent Authority of the exporting country or a certifying official approved by the importing country, and that are accompanied by an international aquatic animal health certificate.

Sections 1.6 and 1.7 provide guidelines for "Contingency plans" and for "Fallowing in aquaculture", respectively.

Part 2 of the Aquatic Code

Part 2 contains recommendations for diseases of fish, molluscs and crustaceans, respectively. The recommendations are designed to minimise the risk of the disease under consideration being introduced and established in the importing country, taking into account the nature of the traded commodity and the aquatic animal health status of the exporting country. This means that, correctly applied, the recommendations ensure that the intended importation can take place with an optimal level of animal health security, incorporating the latest scientific findings and available techniques.

Disease chapters are presented in a consistent format. Article 1is on the definition of the disease for the purposes of the *Aquatic Code*. Article 2 is on the scope of the chapter, *i.e.*, those host species that are susceptible to the disease in question and are internationally traded.

Article 3 in conjunction with Articles 7 to 12 contain recommendations for the trade of "safe" commodities; when authorising import or transit, Competent Authorities should not require any conditions relating to the disease in question, regardless of the status of the exporting country, zone or compartment for that disease. (This concept was introduced to provide better guidance to OIE Member Countries on commodities that can be traded safely and also to better reflect the realities of trade, e.g., the fact that more than 90% of the 50 million tonnes live weight equivalent of world fish production traded internationally in 2002 was in processed form [2]). For all other commodities, consistent with the SPS Agreement, importing countries should not simply reject a commodity because it is deemed "too risky." Rather, importing countries should assess the risk and try to manage it down to an acceptable level. To aid this process, guidance is provided on disease-specific risk management measures that depend on the status of the exporting country, zone or compartment for that disease and also take into account the intended end-use for the traded commodity (for example, release into aquaculture, or direct human consumption).

Articles 4, 5 and 6 are on self-declaration of freedom (country, zone and compartment), and for maintaining and regaining freedom. Three different pathways are described: the absence of susceptible species; historical freedom; and targeted surveillance with negative results (to be underpinned with scientifically based, disease-specific surveys). This constitutes a graded, risk-based approach. For example, where there are no susceptible species, there is no need for targeted surveillance, but basic biosecurity conditions need to be in place before the country, zone or compartment may be declared free. These basic biosecurity conditions are defined in the *Aquatic Code*. They require, inter alia, that an early detection system is in place that must include "*veterinarians or aquatic animal health specialists trained in recognising and reporting suspicious disease occurrence*".

The OIE *Manual of Diagnostic Tests for Aquatic Animals*

The aim of the *Aquatic Manual* is to provide a uniform approach to the diagnosis of the diseases listed in the *Aquatic Code* and of other diseases that may be of importance to trade, so that the requirements for health certification in connection with trade in aquatic animals and aquatic animal products can be met. This is achieved through the detailing of pathogen identification methods that are suitable for the diagnosis of isolated cases of disease as part of national aquatic animal health surveillance or control programmes, or as part of a programme to underpin claims of freedom from a specific disease.

The *Aquatic Manual* is updated regularly, and a new edition is published every two to three years in hard copy and on-line [3]. More frequent updates (in highlighted format) are made to the on-line version. Part 1 of the *Aquatic Manual* contains general provisions, while Part 2 details recommendations applicable to specific diseases. In Part 3, the list of OIE Reference Laboratories and Collaborating Centres for diseases of fish, molluscs and crustaceans is provided.

Part 1 of the Aquatic Manual

Chapter 1.1.1. is about quality management in veterinary testing laboratories. Chapter 1.1.2. explains the principles of validation of diagnostic assays for infectious diseases, and Chapter 1.1.3. provides guidance specifically for the validation and quality control of polymerase chain reaction methods. Chapter 1.1.4. describes the requirements for surveillance for declaration of freedom from infection. Chapter 1.1.5. details methods for disinfection of aquaculture establishments.

Part 2 of the Aquatic Manual

Part 2 contains recommendations for diseases of fish, molluscs and crustaceans, respectively. Disease chapters are presented in a consistent format that links back to the corresponding chapters in the *Aquatic Code*. Section 1 is on case definitions. Section 2 is on information for the design of surveillance programmes: agent factors, *e.g.*, aetiological agent, agent strains, survival outside the host, and stability; host factors, *e.g.*, susceptible species and their stages, target organs and infected tissue, and vectors; disease pattern, *e.g.*, occurrence and transmission mechanisms, prevalence, geographical distribution, mortality and morbidity, and economic and/or production impact; and control and prevention, *e.g.*, vaccination, chemotherapy, immunostimulation, resistance breeding, restocking with resistant species, blocking agents, and general husbandry practices.

Section 3 is on diagnostic methods: field methods; clinical methods; and agent detection and identification methods, *e.g.*, direct detection methods (microscopic methods, agent isolation and identification through cell culture/artificial media, antibody-based antigen detection methods, and molecular techniques) and indirect methods (serology).

Section 4 is on rating of tests against purpose of use. Section 5 looks at corroborative diagnostic criteria with the definition of a suspect and confirmed case. Section 6 lays out diagnostic/detection methods to declare freedom.

OIE Reference Laboratories and Collaborating Centres

There are currently 27 OIE Reference Laboratories for aquatic animal diseases. Under the guidance of an expert whose competence is recognised internationally, they function as centres of expertise and standardisation of diagnostic techniques. They may also provide scientific and technical training for personnel from Member Countries, and coordinate scientific and technical studies in collaboration with other laboratories or organisations.

The OIE Collaborating Centre for Information on Aquatic Diseases is located in Weymouth in the UK. It developed and maintains an international database on aquatic animal disease occurrence that is freely available via the internet (www.collabcen.net). This database can also be accessed through the Aquatic Animals Commission's web pages. The Director of the Collaborating Centre is also the chief editor for the Aquatic Animals Commission's web pages. These pages provide technical information on aquatic animal health issues and a "latest news" service (www.oie.int/aac/eng/en_fdc.htm).

Raising Awareness about Aquatic Animal Health

The OIE is committed to raising awareness about aquatic animal health and assisting Member Countries to discharge their international obligations. Supported by the OIE Central Bureau, members of the Aquatic Animals Commission regularly present on the activities of the Aquatic Animals Commission at the (mostly biannual) Conferences of the OIE's five Regional Commissions (Africa; the Americas; Asia, the Far East and Oceania; Europe; and the Middle East). Next to Commission members, the OIE Director General himself uses the opportunity these Conferences provide to remind Delegates to continue implementing the "Nouméa Recommendations", a set of recommendations aimed at, *inter alia*, improving cooperation between veterinary and other competent authorities on aquatic animal health matters. (The "Nouméa Recommendations" had been adopted by the OIE Regional Commission for Asia, the Far East and Oceania on 28 November, 2003, and subsequently endorsed by the International Committee of the OIE on 27 May, 2004 [4]).

Aquatic Animals Commission members make presentations and hold workshops at scientific conferences. Examples of conferences from the last few years include the International Symposium on Veterinary Epidemiology and Economics (2003); the World Aquaculture Society Special Session on Biosecurity (March 2004); the Sixth Symposium on Diseases in Asian Aquaculture (Oct 2005); the International Forum on Infectious Myonecrosis in farmed shrimp (August 2006); the First Global Conference on Aquatic Animal Health (2006); and the First International Conference of OIE Reference Laboratories and Collaborating Centres (2006).

The Aquatic Animals Commission provides a permanent member to the Asia-Pacific Regional Advisory Group on Aquatic Animal Health. This group was established by the Governing Council of the Network of Aquaculture Centres in Asia-Pacific (NACA) to provide advice to NACA members in the Asia-Pacific region on aquatic animal health management. Next to the Aquatic Animals Commission representative, members of the Advisory Group include invited aquatic animal disease experts, the OIE Regional Representation for Asia and the Pacific, FAO, and collaborating regional organisations. The group has met annually since 2002 and continues to, *inter alia*, review the regional aquatic animal disease status and assess and make recommendations for regional aquatic animal disease reporting. It also assists in improving cooperation between veterinary and fisheries authorities in the region. The group's comprehensive reports are published on the NACA website http://www.enaca.org/. Aquatic Animals Commission members also engage in FAO expert consultations, for example on surveillance, monitoring and zoning in 2002 [5] and, more recently in 2005, on responsible introductions and movement of live aquatics [6].

Challenges Ahead

Over the past few years, new topics have arisen for the OIE in the field of aquatic animals, for example aquatic animal welfare, and the development of antimicrobial resistance in aquaculture. The safety of aquatic feeds for aquatic animals is another novel topic that requires detailed consideration before recommendations can be developed for the *Aquatic Code*.

Unlike the terrestrial animal farming sector which relies on a comparatively small number of usually well-domesticated animals worldwide, aquaculture continues to trial "new" species for their suitability to breed and grow under controlled conditions. Typically, little is known about the health status of such new candidate species, their nutritional and other husbandry requirements, or – indeed – their life cycle. Frequently, broodstock are taken from the wild, increasing the risk of introducing pathogens into hatcheries. New diseases therefore continue to emerge, and developing diagnostic techniques is a "catch-up" game.

Multi-agent disease syndromes are common in the aquatic environment and are increasingly described particularly in crustacean hosts. Since most crustacean viruses cannot yet be grown in cell culture, infectivity trials are hampered severely and it is difficult to ascertain which role – if any – a particular infectious agent plays in the syndrome. This is far from being an academic or research problem; rather, it severely compromises the development of case definitions for disease reporting purposes and the development of control strategies.

Finally, the OIE will need to decide whether it wishes to further expand its remit to cover diseases of amphibians and reptiles.

References

1 World Organisation for Animal Health: *OIE Aquatic Animal Health Code*. Paris, France, 9th edition, 2006. (Accessed 2 January 2007 from http://www.oie.int/eng/normes/fcode/en_sommaire.htm).

2 FAO: The State of World Fisheries and Aquaculture. Food and Agriculture Organization of the United Nations. Rome, Italy, 2004. (Accessed 2 January 2007 from http://www.fao.org/documents/show_cdr.asp?url_file=/DOCREP/007/y5600e/y5600e00.htm).

3 World Organisation for Animal Health: *OIE Manual of Diagnostic Tests for Aquatic Animals*. Paris, 5th edition, 2006. (Accessed 2 January 2007 from http://www.oie.int/eng/normes/fmanual/A_summry.htm).

4 23rd Conference of the OIE Regional Commission for Asia, the Far East and Oceania, Nouméa (New Caledonia), 25-28 November 2003: Recommendation No. 2: Update on developments in aquatic animal diseases, in OIE: Final Report 2004. 72nd General Session, Paris, 23-28 May 2004. OIE, Paris, 2004, pp 169-171. (Accessed 22 December 2006 from http://www.oie.int/eng/OIE/actes/en_rfinal.htm).

5 Subasinghe RP, McGladdery SE, Hill BJ (eds): Surveillance and zoning for aquatic animal diseases. FAO Fisheries Technical Paper. No. 451. Rome, FAO. 2004. (Accessed 2 January 2007 from http://www.fao.org/docrep/007/y5325e/y5325e00.htm).

6 FAO: Aquaculture development. 2. Health management for responsible movement of live aquatic animals. FAO Technical Guidelines for Responsible Fisheries. No. 5. Rome, FAO. 2007.

Dr. Eva-Maria Bernoth, Dr med vet, President, OIE Aquatic Animal Health Standards Commission, c/o Office of the Chief Veterinary Officer, Australian Government Department of Agriculture, Fisheries and Forestry, GPO Box 858, Canberra ACT 2601, Australia
E-mail: Eva-Maria.Bernoth@daff.gov.au

Dodet B, the OIE Scientific & Technical Department (eds): The OIE Global Conference on Aquatic Animal Health. Dev Biol (Basel). Basel, Karger, 2007, vol 129, p 171.

Session VII

Conference Recommendations and the Way Forward

Chairperson: *T. Håstein*, Norway

Dodet B, the OIE Scientific & Technical Department (eds): The OIE Global Conference on Aquatic Animal Health. Dev Biol (Basel). Basel, Karger, 2007, vol 129, pp 173-175.

Recommendations

THE OIE GLOBAL CONFERENCE ON AQUATIC ANIMAL HEALTH

CONSIDERING THAT,

- Aquaculture production now provides over forty per cent of the total world production of aquatic animals for human consumption.
- Aquatic animal diseases are a major constraint for production and trade.
- An increasing number of species are farmed worldwide, but few are domesticated; hence there is inadequate knowledge about the health status and disease control of many farmed species.
- In many Member Countries, aquatic animal health management is a responsibility that is shared among several authorities and the private sector.
- Legislation and regulatory frameworks have been successfully implemented in some Member Countries, sometimes with monitoring and control procedures in place as well as legal action for non-compliance.
- In many countries, there is a need for improving governance and capacity building (institutions, policy, and legal frameworks) in aquatic animal health management.
- Investment in aquatic animal health can be highly variable and often does not reflect the value and volume of the commodities produced.
- Organising and empowering farmers (particularly in small-scale farming operations) and application of better management practices could effectively reduce losses due to diseases in aquaculture.
- In preparing the national infrastructure for disease surveillance and emergency response, it is crucial to share expertise, ownership, resources, information and vision among stakeholders.
- Communication, co-operation and co-ordination play paramount roles in aquatic animal health management and disease emergency preparedness.
- Timely and accurate reporting of disease events is essential for transparency and for strengthening the confidence of Member Countries in the aquatic animal health status of their trading partners; countries that do not respect international aquatic animal disease reporting obligations can be a threat to their trading partners.

- Education is a pillar in aquatic animal health management; specialised training is available, but existing education systems can be too slow to address emerging needs.
- Students' and professionals' needs are evolving, which requires a variety of programmes and flexible teaching methods.
- With reduced government funding for training and education, there is a need for industry to contribute.
- For most Member Countries, aquatic animal welfare is a new initiative; future international standards and guidelines should be based on sound science and include performance indicators.
- Farming slaughter practices have originated from traditional fisheries.
- With respect to aquatic animal welfare, cultural differences among Member Countries are important, and all Member Countries have the opportunity to comment on the draft guidelines.

THE PARTICIPANTS IN THE OIE GLOBAL CONFERENCE ON AQUATIC ANIMAL HEALTH

RECOMMEND THAT,

1. Within Member Countries:

a) there be a dialogue among the veterinary authorities, other relevant authorities, and the private sector, to identify their respective roles and responsibilities in aquatic animal health management;

b) a regulatory framework for aquatic animal health be established, and enforcement of law and implementation of regulatory procedures be strengthened;

c) national aquatic animal health strategies be prepared. Such strategies should:

    i. be capable of dealing with ongoing challenges and be responsive to changing demands;
    ii. use available resources, even if they are limited;
    iii. take on board relevant experiences;
    iv. promote ownership by all relevant stakeholders and clarify responsibilities to maximise compliance;
    v. clarify mechanisms for funding, communication and implementation;
    vi. address disease prevention and control, e.g. through appropriate contingency plans that ensure emergency readiness and provide the ability to build up resources quickly and effectively; and
    vii. include clear command structures;

d) accuracy and timeliness of aquatic animal disease reports be significantly improved, and the OIE's assistance requested where clarification is needed.

2. And that the OIE provide Member Countries with the necessary assistance and guidance on accurate, timely and effective aquatic animal disease reporting, and continue to:

a) provide opportunities for cooperation between veterinary and other authorities and the private sector responsible for aquatic animal health in Member Countries;

b) direct efforts at increasing general awareness with national Delegates world-wide about the provisions of the Aquatic Code and Aquatic Manual;

c) encourage Member Countries to strengthen veterinary and other tertiary education in aquatic animal health as well as practical training for farmers;

d) cooperate with relevant international and regional organisations to increase awareness about aquatic animal health, to improve disease reporting and to foster cooperation between veterinary and other relevant authorities within Member Countries and between international organisations; and

e) work, through its Animal Welfare Working Group and other relevant international fora, on aquatic animal welfare.

Dodet B, the OIE Scientific & Technical Department (eds): The OIE Global Conference on Aquatic Animal Health. Dev Biol (Basel). Basel, Karger, 2007, vol 129, p 177-178.

Closing Remarks

We have now had two days full of comprehensive presentations and enlightening discussions on a pressing issue that is very important for all of us. Together we have done great work here, intensively; we probably could have gone on for another two days.

What were our objectives?

We talked about helping to build a framework for improved involvement and cooperation between the involved authorities, the scientific community and the private sector; helping to clarify roles and responsibilities of all stakeholders; helping increase aquatic animal health emergency response capability; exchanging information on emerging diseases and animal welfare issues and helping to develop a science based approach to the management of aquatic animal health and welfare.

We have actually managed to touch on all these issues and present some important and relevant recommendations that the OIE Aquatic Animal Health Commission should further develop as part of their excellent work.

I would like to give some personal recommendations based upon some the very good presentations and comments I have heard here over these two days. I would like you all to help spread the message when you go back home. Make contact, communicate and build partnerships to emphasize the importance of putting resources into this field, into planning, information dissemination and capacity building and training concerning aquatic animal health and welfare so that the next time we meet we may say we are better prepared for both the expected and the unexpected diseases or issues. Do not wait for more resources, try to make the best out of what you have.

The OIE has a remit and responsibility for aquatic animal diseases and welfare, but the OIE is no better than the sum of its Member Countries. We must all assume our responsibility to contribute to this important issue.

I am sure the OIE aquatic animal health commission will continue to spread the word through the networks of regional and sub-regional offices of the OIE, and through good cooperation with other international and regional organisations such as FAO and the NACA. The OIE is also planning a future Scientific Review on aquatic animal health and welfare that will also present some important presentations as a follow-up to this conference.

Finally, remember to focus on the critical success criteria of communication, coordination and cooperation.

Thank you for a fruitful conference and continue your untiring efforts in this field when you get back home.

Dr. Keren Bar-Yaacov,
Chief Veterinary Officer

List of Participants

••••••••••••••••••

AARFLOT Leiv, Nedre Bergslia 8 Fosnavåg , N-6090 Norway

AFONSO Ana, Polyviou Scientific Panel on Animal Health and Welfare European Food Safety Authority Largo N. Palli 5/A, 43100 Parma - ITALY

AL SUNUAIHER Anwar, P.O. Box 275 Riyadh 11311 Saudi Arabia

AMOS Kevin, National Fish Health Co-ordinator, NOAA/NMFS, U.S. Dept. of Commerce, 8924 Libby RD NE, Olympia, WA 98506, USA BARROS CAVALCANTE José, Ministério da Agricultura, Pecuária e Abastecimento, Esplanada dos Ministérios - Bloco D - Anexo A - Sala 308 - CEP: 70.043-900 - Brasilia – DF

BATHO Howard, European Commission, Rue Froissart 101 Brussels , 1049 Belgium

BERGERSEN Bente, The Norwegian Food Safety Authority, National Fish and Seafood Centre, Rosenkrantzgate 3, 5003 Bergen, Norway

BERLINGIERI Francesco

BHATTACHARRY Ajay, Department of Animal Husbandry Dairying and Fisheries Ministry of AgricultureKrishi Bhavan, New Delhi 110001, India

BJORLOW Inge, The Norwegian Food Safety Langg. 1D Sandnes, 4306 Norway

BLAIR Marilyn, USFWS Idaho Fish Health CenterP.O. Box 272 Orofino, ID 83544

BOVO Giuseppe, Istituto Zooprofilattico Sperimentale delle Venezie Viale Dell'Universita'10 Legnaro (PD) 35020 Italy

BRUN Edgar, National Veterinary Institute, PO Box 8156 Dep Oslo, 033, Norway

BRUNDTLAND Marthe

BRUNVOLD Laila, Institute of Marine Research, P.O. Box 1870 Nordnes, NO-5817 Bergen, Norway

CAPUANO Donatella, Ministero della Salute Direzione Generale Sanità animale e farmaco veterinario Ufficio VIII Piazzale Marconi 25 00144 Rome, Italy

CHAISEMARTIN Daniel, World Organisation for Animal Health (OIE) 12, rue de Prony 75017 Paris, France

CHENG CHUNG Leo, GeneReach Biotechnology Corp.No. 2-1, 7th Road,Taichung Industrial Park Taichung 407 Taiwan

CORSIN Flavio, Network of Aquaculture Centres in Asia-Pacific (NACA) c/o NAFIQAVED, Ministry of Fisheries Ba Dinh District, Ha Noi Viet Nam

DALTVEIT Magnhild, Mattilsynet DK Sunnhordland Felles Postmottak Postboks 383, 2381 Brumunddal Brumunddal, 1 2381 Norway

DAVENPORT Keith, Ornamental Aquatic Trade Association Ltd (OATA), 1st Floor Office Suite, Wessex House, 40 Station Road, Westbury, Wiltshire, BA13 3JN, UK

DE AZEVEDO PEDROSA CUNHA Eduardo , Esplanada dos Ministérios, Bloco D, CEP: 70043-900 CTQA/DSA/SDA/MAPA Sala 322 A, Brasília, DF Brasil

DIEMER Michael

DJUPEVIK Hans Olav, Norwegian Food Safety Authority, Djupvik, 5641 Fusa, Norway EITHUN Inger, Norwegian Food Safety Authority, Felles postmottak, Pb 383, Brumunddal, Norway

ENRIQUEZ Ricardo FARSTAD Wenche, Professor, DVM dr.scient, PhDDipl ECAR Norwegian School of Veterinary Science Department of Production Anmal Clinical Sciences P.O.Box 8146 DEp, N-0033 Oslo, Norway

FERNANDEZ Peter, US Mission to the EU, blvd du Regent 27 Brussels, 1000 Belgium

FLATNES Myklebust Cecilie, Ministry of Fisheries and Coastal affairs PO Box 8118 Dep Oslo, 0032 Norway

FORWARD Benjamin, The New Brunswick Research & Productivity Council, 921 College Hill Rd, Fredericton, New Brunswick, Canada

FOSSA Svein A., Norges Zoohandleres Bransjeforening Fladefjell 15 Grimstad, NO-4878 Norway

FRANCOIS Cyrill, Avenue de Mus de loup, 17390 La Tremblade, France

FYLLINGEN Inger, P.O. Box 2009 Nordnes NO -5817 Bergen Norway GEOGHEGAN Fiona, Fish Health Unit, Marine Institute, Rinville, Oranmore, Co. Galway, Ireland

GUDDING Roar, Roar Gudding National veterianry Institute POBox 8156 Dep 0033 Oslo Norway

GUICHARD Benjamin, AFSSA-ANMV Unité Evaluation des Médicaments Chimiques, BP 90203, La Haute Marche, Javené 35302 Fougères France

GUTIERREZ Jesus

GUZMAN Nimer, Calle José Natusch N° 271 Santísima Trinidad Beni - Bolivia HAMMELL K. Larry, University of Prince Edward Island 550 University Avenue Charlottetown, PEI , C1A 4P3 Canada

HASTEIN Tore, Senior rådgiver/senior advisor Veterinærinstituttet/National Veterinary Institute PO box 8156 DEP N-0033 Oslo, Norway

HASTINGS Trevor, FRS Marine Laboratory 375 Victoria Road Aberdeen AB11 9DB, Scotland, UK

HELLBERG Hege, National Veterinary Institute, P.O. Box 1263 Sentrum, 5811 Bergen, Norway

HELLSTROM Anders, National Veterinary Institute Avdelningen för vilt, fisk och miljö/Department of wildlife, fish and environment 751 89 Uppsala, Sweden

HINEY Maura, National University of Ireland, IT Building, NUI Galway, Galway City, Ireland

HOLM Jens Christian, Aquaculture and Coastal Management Dept. Directorate of Fisheries, .O. Box 2009 Nordnes,NO-5817 Bergen Norway

HOUSE Nancy, National Registry of Aquatic Animal Health Fisheries and Oceans Canada 200, rue Kent St.12W114, Ottawa, ON K1A 0E6 CANADA

HUNG Le Dinh, Ministry of Fisheries of Vietnam 10 Nguyen Cong Hoan, Ba Dinh District, Hanoi

IIDA Takaji, Aquatic Animal Health Division, National Research Institute of Aquaculture, Fisheries Research Agency, Minami-Ise, Mie 516-0193, Japan

JENSEN Pal Erik

JIANG Yulin, The Key Lab of Aquatic Animal Diseases Shenzhen Exit&entry Inspection and Quarantine Bureau B801 Heping Building, 2049 Heping Road, Shenzhen, 518001 China

JOHANSEN Renate, Norwegian school of veterinary science P. box 8146 dep0033 Oslo Norway

JOHNSEN Stian, Mattilsynet/ Norwegian Food Safety Authority, hovedkontoretPostboks 383, 2381 Brummundal, Oslo, Norway KANCHANAKHAN Somkiat, Inland Aquatic Animal Health Research Institute (AAHRI) Inland Fisheries Research and Development Bureau Department of Fisheries Paholyothin Road, Jatuchak Bangkok 10900, Thailand

KANG Jaeyoun, Quality management division National Fisheries Products Quality Inspection Service. 192-7 Ilsan 2 dong, Ilsan gu, Koyang si, Kyunggi do, Republic of Korea (410-315)

KARATAS Suheyla, Istanbul University Fisheries Faculty Ordu Cad. No:200 34470 Laleli Istanbul, Turkey

KARREMAN Grace, Pacific Marine Veterinary Services 3000 Andre Road Nanaimo, BC V9R 6X2 Canada

KIBENGE Frederick, Atlantic Veterinary College, University of Prince Edward Island, Department of Pathology and Microbiology Atlantic Veterinary Cellege, UPEI 550 University Avenue Charlott Etown, PEI C1A 4P3, Canada, Charlott Etown, Canada

KORSNES Kjetil, Post box 1870 Nordnes Bergen 5817 Norway

LARSSEN Rolf.B., Norwegian School of Veterinary Science POB 8146 Ullevalsvn 72, Oslo NO 0033 Norway

LAVILLA PITOGO Celia, Southeast Asian Fisheries Development, Center - Aquaculture Department Tigbauan 5021, Iloilo, Philippines

LE DUY Binh, Le Duy Binh 30 Ham Nghi street, District 1, Ho chi Minh City, Viet Nam

LE GROUMELLEC Marc, Nicole Le Groumellec 3, Impasse Des Fusains 56260 Larmor-Plage France

LEE Sangyoon, National Fisheries Products Quality Inspection Service Incheon branch 30-16 Shinheung-dong 3ga, joong-gu, Incheon-si, Republic of Korea (400-103)

LEON Pilar, Subdirección General de Ordenación y Buenas Prácticas Ganaderas.C/ Alfonso XII 62. 28014 Madrid España.

LIGHTNER Donald, Aquaculture Pathology Laboratory, Department of Veterinary Science and Microbiology, University of Arizona, Building 90, Room 202 Pharmacy/Microbiology, Tucson, AZ 85721, USA

LILLEAAS Bjarne M., Felles Postmottak Postboks 383 2381 Brumunddal Brumunddal, 2381 Norway

LILLEHAUG Atle, National Veterinary Institute PO Box 8156 Dep. N-0033 Oslo Norway

LIU Hong, The Key Lab of Aquatic Animal Diseases Shenzhen Exit&entry Inspection and Quarantine Bureau B801 Heping Building, 2049 Heping Road, Shenzhen 518001 China

LO Grace Chu-Fang, No.1, Sec. 4, Roosevelt Rd ROC Lab of Crustacean Virology, Institute of Zoology, NTU - Room 818, Life Science Building Taipei 106 Taiwan

LOPEZ DORIGA Victoria, Schering-Plough Ltd Breakspear Road South Harefield Uxbridge Middlesex UB9 6LS UK

LYONS Mary Maille MALTSEV Vyacheslav, Zonal Specialized State Laboratory of Veterinary Medicine, Relative to Diseases of Fishes and other Aquatic Animals, 65, Furmanov Str., Kerch, Crimea, Ukraine, 98300

MANFRIN Amedeo, Laboratorio di Adria Via L. da Vinci, 39 45011 Adria, Roma, Italy

MARTINS Serzants

MATRAS Marek

MELHUUS Brynjulf, Ullevålsveien 76 Oslo Box 383,2381 Brumunddal Norway

MELINGEN Geir Olav, Schering-Plough Animal Health Ankerveien 209 1359 Eiksmarka, Norway

MELSTOKKA Maria, Norwegian Food Safety Authority Rosenkrantzgate 3 Bergen, 5003 Norway

MILLER Otis, 12021 Jasmine Cove Way Raleigh, NC 27614 USA

MORTENSEN Stein, Institute of Marine Research Nordnesgt 50, Nordnes Bergen ,5817 Norway

MULLIN David, Fish Health Unit Defra (VEROD Team G) Area 108 1A Page Street London SW 1P 4PQ UK

MURRAY Alexander G.: Fisheries Research Services Marine Laboratory, 375 Victoria Road, Aberdeen, UK

MYKLEBUST Cecilie Flatnes O'BRIEN Nicole, NL DFA - Aquaculture Health Unit Aquaculture Veterinarian 30 Strawberry Marsh Road Petten Building PO Box 8700 St. John's, NL Canada A1B 4J6

OLESEN Niels Jorgen, Danish institute for Food and Veterinary Research Hangøvej 2 DK-8200 Århus N Denmark

OLSEN Anne - Berit, National Veterinary Institute Bergen P.O. Box 1263 Sentrum Bergen, 5811 Norway

ORAIC Drazen, Croatian Veterinary Institute Dept. of Fish Diseases and Aquaculture Savska 143, 10000 Zagreb, Croatia

ORMSETTROE Stein Ivar

PALIC Dusan, Center for Food Security and Public Health, The College of Veterinary Medicine, Iowa State University, 2160 College of Veterinary Medicine, Ames, Iowa, USA

RAHKONEN Ritta, Ministry of Agriculture and Forestry, Department of Food and Health, PO Box 30, Helsinki FI-00023, Finland

RAYNARD Robert, Fisheries Research Services Marine Laboratory PO Box 101 375 Victoria Road Aberdeen, AB11 9DB, UK

REANTASO Melba, NACA,Suraswadi Building, Department of Fisheries Compound, Kasetsart University Campu, Ladyao, Jatujak, Bangkok, Thailand

RICHARDS Randolph, Institute of Aquaculture University of Stirling Stirling, FK9 4LA, UK

ROLLAND Jill, Aquaculture Specialist USDA/APHIS/VS/ASEP 4700 River Road, Unit 46, 4B-02.5 Riverdale, MD 20737 SANCHEZ SANCHEZ Celia, Subdirección General de Ordenación y Buenas Prácticas Ganaderas. C/ Alfonso XII 62.28014 Madrid, Spain.

SANDLUND Nina, Institute of Marine Research P.O box 1870 Nordnes Bergen, NO-5817 Norway

SCARFE David, AVMA, PO Box 6100, Mississippi States, MS 39762, USA

SCUDAMORE Jim, 56 Horseshoe Lane East Guildford GU1 2TL, UK

SLAATTO NAESS Ingfrid, Norwegian Scientific Committee for Food Safety v/Ingfrid Slaatto Næss P.O. Box 4404 Nydalen N-0403 Oslo, Norway

SNOW Michael, FRS Marine Laboratory Aberdeen,FRS Marine Laboratory 375 Victoria Rd Aberdeen AB11 9DB, Aberdeen, Scotland

STANIFORD Don, Spinney House, St. David's Lane, NoctorumBirkenhead, Merseyside, CH43 9UD, UK

STRAUME-LIE Kristian, Mattilsynet Regionkontor for Hordaland, Sogn og Fjordane Rosenkrantzgate 3 2003 Bergen, Norway

SUBASINGHE Rohana, Senior Fishery Resources Officer Fisheries Department Food and Agriculture Organization of the UN Viale delle Terme di Caracalla 00100 Rome, Italy

SUNDE Irja Roiha, Institute of Marine Research Postboks 1870, Nordnes Bergen, N-5817 Norway

SUZUKI Takashi, Japan Apan Fisheries Resource Conservattion Association West 303-2, 2-18-1 Kachidoki, Chuo-ku, Tokyo, 104-0054, Japan

SVERDRUP Anne, Thormøhlensgate 55 Bergen, 5008 Norway TELES-GRILO Maria Leonor, Instituto de Ciências Biomédicas Abel Salazar - Universidade do Porto Largo Prof Abel Salazar, nº2 Porto , 4099-003 Portugal

TOPS Sylvie, Schering-Plough Animal Health, Breakspear Road South, Harefield, Uxbridge, Middlesex UB9 6LS, U.K.

TORGERSEN Yngve, Deputy Director General Ministry of Fisheries and Coastal Affairs P.o.Box 8118 Dep, N-0032 Oslo, Norway

TORRES Pilar, Laboratorio Central de Veterinaria Ctra. de Algete, km. 8 28110 Algete, Madrid, Spain

ULVENES Marianne, Grasmenipo 29 5355 Knrarrevik, Norway VAZQUEZ JUAREZ Ricardo, CIBNOR Mar bermejo 195 Col Playa Palo Santa Rita La Paz Baja California, 23090 Mexico

VESELEY Tomas, Veterinary Research Institute, 62100 Brno, Czech Republic

VIGO MARTIN Marta, Laboratorio Central de Veterinaria Ctra. de Algete, km. 8 28110 Algete, Madrid, Spain WAAGBO Rune,NIFES (National Institute ok Nutrition and Seafood Research), NIFES, PO Box 2029 Nordnes, 5817 Bergen, Norway

WALKER Peter, Australian Animal Health Laboratory, CSIRO Livestock Industries, 5 Portarlington Road, Geelong VIC 3220, Australia

WANG Han Ching, No. 1, Sec. 4, Roosevelt Road Taipei, 10617 Taiwan

WARG Janet, Diagnostic Virology Laboratory National Veterinary Services Laboratories P. O. Box 844 Ames, Iowa 50010 USA

WEIMER Udo, Bundesministerium für ernährung, landwirtschaft und Verbraucherschutz Rochusstraße 1 Bonn, 53123 Germany

WHELAN Daryl, Provincial Aquaculture Veterinarian Aquaculture Health Unit, PO Box 8700 30 Strawberry Marsh Road, Petten Bldg.St. John's, NL Canada A1B 4J6

WICHARDT Ulf Peter, Fish Health Control Programme Uppsalavagen 3 SE-814 70 Alvkarleby, Sweden

YOSHIMIZU Mamoru, Graduate School of Fisheries Science, Hokkaido University, Hokkaido 041-8611, Japan

ZRNCIC Snježana, Croatian Veterinary Institute Dept. of Fish Diseases Savska 143, 10000 Zagreb, Croatia

Index of Authors

Developments in Biological Standardization

Vol. 36	Washington DC, 1976	Freeze-Drying of Biological Products
Vol. 37	Geneva, 1976	Standardization of Cell Substrates for the Production of Virus Vaccines
Vol. 38	London, 1977	Biological Preparations in the Treatment of Cancer
Vol. 39	Geneva, 1977	Influenza Immunization
Vol. 40	Marburg, 1977	Standardization of Rabies Vaccines for Human Use Produced in Tissue Culture (Rabies III)
Vol. 41	Guadeloupe, 1978	Vaccines in the Developing Countries
Vol. 42	Paris, 1978	Second General Meeting of ESACT
Vol. 43	Brussels, 1978	Immunization: Benefit Versus Risk Factors
Vol. 44	Villars, 1979	Test methods for the Quality Control of Plasma Proteins
Vol. 45	San Antonio, 1979	The Standardization of Animals to Improve Biomedical Research, Production and Control
Vol. 46	Oxford, 1979	Third General Meeting of ESACT
Vol. 47	Bilthoven, 1980	Reassessment of Inactivated Poliomyelitis Vaccine
Vol. 48	Geneva, 1980	Standardization of Albumin, Plasma Substitutes and Plasmapheresis
Vol. 49	Leetown, 1981	Fish Biologics: Serodiagnostics and Vaccines
Vol. 50	Heidelberg, 1981	The Use of Heteroploid and Other Cell Substrates for the Production of Biologicals
Vol. 51	Lyons, 1981	Immunization of Adult Birds with Inactivated Oil Adjuvant Vaccines
Vol. 52	Lyons, 1981	Herpes Virus of Man and Animal: Standardization of Immunological Procedures
Vol. 53	Dublin, 1982	Enteric Infections in Man and Animals: Standardization of Immunological Procedures
Vol. 54	Athens, 1982	Viral Hepatitis: Standardization in Immunoprophylaxis of Infections by Hepatitis Viruses
Vol. 55	Copenhagen, 1982	Fifth General Meeting of ESCAT
Vol. 56	Algiers, 1983	Third International Symposium on Brucellosis
Vol. 57	Paris, 1983	Monoclonal Antibodies: Standardization of their Characterization and Use
Vol. 58	Budapest, 1983	International Symposium on BCG Vaccines and Tuberculins
Vol. 59	Geneva, 1983	Standardization and Control of Biologicals Produced by Recombinant DNA Technology
Vol. 60	Gardone Riviera, 1984	Production and Exploitation of Existing and New Animal Cell Sub strates
Vol. 61	Geneva, 1984	Proceedings of the Fourth International Symposium on Pertussis
Vol. 62	Stockholm, 1985	Diagnostics and Vaccines for Parasitic Diseases
Vol. 63	San Francisco, 1985	Use and Standardization of Chemically Defined Antigens
Vol. 64	London, 1985	Reduction of Animal Usage in the Development and Control of Biological Products
Vol. 65	Amsterdam, 1985	Use and Standardization of Combined Vaccines

Vol. 66	Vienna, 1985	Advances in Animal Cell Technology: Cell Engineering, Evaluation and Exploitation
Vol. 67	Melbourne, 1986	Standardization in Blood Fractionation Including Coagulation Factors
Vol. 68	Geneva, 1986	Cells - Products - Safety
Vol. 69	London, 1987	Cytokines Laboratory and Clinical Evaluation
Vol. 70	Arlington, VA, 1988	Continuous Cell Lines as Substrates for Biologicals
Vol. 71	Utrecht, 1989	Monoclonal Antibodies for Therapy, Prevention and In vivo Diagnosis of Human Disease
Vol. 72	Annecy, 1989	Progress in Animal Retroviruses
Vol. 73	Shizuoka, 1990	Pertussis: Evaluation and Research on Acellular Pertussis Vaccines
Vol. 74	Bethesda, MD, 1990	Biological Product Freeze-Drying and Formulation
Vol. 75	London, 1990	Virological Aspects of the Safety of Biological Products
Vol. 76	Bethesda, MD, 1991	Continuous Cell Lines - An International Workshop on Current Issues
Vol. 77	Annecy, 1991	Standardization of the Immunopharmacology of Natural and Synthetic Immunomodulators
Vol. 78	Bethesda, MD, 1991	Poliovirus Attenuation: Molecular Mechanisms and Practical Aspects
Vol. 79	Ploufragan, 1992	The First Steps Towards an International Harmonization of Veterinary Biologicals: 1993 and Free Circulation of Vaccines within the EEC
Vol. 80	Heidelberg, 1992	Transmissible Spongiform Encephalopathies - Impact on Animal and Human Health
Vol. 81	Cannes, 1992	Virological Safety Aspects of Plasma Derivatives
Vol. 82	Albany NY, 1993	Recombinant Vectors in Vaccine Development
Vol. 83	Annecy, 1993	Genetic Stability and Recombinant Product Consistency
Vol. 84	Langen, 1993	Non-Target Effects of Live Vaccines
Vol. 85	Santa Fé, NM, 1994	Genetics of Streptococci, Enterococci and Lactococci
Vol. 86	Langen, 1994	Replacement, Reduction and Refinement of Animal Experiments in
the		Development and Control of Biological Products
Vol. 87	Geneva, 1995	New Approaches to Stabilisation of Vaccines Potency
Vol. 88	Bethesda, MD, 1995	Viral Safety and Evaluation of Viral Clearance from Biopharmaceutical Products
Vol. 89	Rome, 1995	Pertussis Vaccine Trials
Vol. 90	Oslo, 1996	Fish Vaccinology
Vol. 91	San Francisco, CA, 1996	Development of Specifications for Biotechnology Pharmaceuticals Products
Vol. 92	Bergen, 1996	Modulation of the Immune Response to Vaccine Antigens
Vol. 93	Annecy, 1996	Safety of Biological Products Prepared from Mammalian Cell Culture
Vol. 94	Bethesda, MD, 1997	Simian Virus 40 (SV40): A Possible Human Polyomavirus
Vol. 95	Paris, 1997	Preclinical and Clinical Development of New Vaccines
Vol. 96	Washington, DC, 1995	Characterization of Biotechnology Pharmaceutical Products
Vol. 97	London, 1997	Biological Characterization and Assay of Cytokines and Growth Factors
Vol. 98	London, 1997	Inactivated Influenza Vaccines Prepared in Cell Culture
Vol. 99	Strasbourg, 1998	Animal Sera, Animal Sera Derivatives and Substitutes Used in the Manufacture of Pharmaceuticals: Viral Safety and Regulatory Aspects
Vol. 100	Geneva, 1998	A Celebration of 50 Years of Progress in Biological Standardization and Control at WHO
Vol. 101	London, 1998	Alternatives to Animals in the Development and Control of Biological Products for Human and Veterinary Use

Developments in Biologicals

Vol. 102	San Francisco, CA, 1999	Advances in Transfusion Safety
Vol. 103	Annecy, 1999	Physico-Chemical Procedures for the Characterization of Vaccines
Vol. 104	Langen, 1999	Development and Clinical Progress of DNA Vaccines
Vol. 105	Paris, 2000	Progress in Polio Eradication: Vaccine Strategies for the End Game
Vol. 106	Rockville, MD, 2000	Evolving Scientific and Regulatory Perspectives on Cell Substrates for Vaccine Development
Vol. 107	London, 2000	The Design and Analysis of Potency Assays for Biotechnology Products
Vol. 108	Langen, 2001	Advances in Transfusion Safety
Vol. 109	Washington, DC, 2000	Biologics 2000 – Comparability of Biotechnology Products
Vol. 110	Palm Cove, 2001	Orphan Vaccines – Bridging the Gap
Vol. 111	Utrecht, 2001	Advancing Science and Elimination of the Use of Laboratory Animals for Development and Control of Vaccines and Hormones
Vol. 112	Bethesda, MD, 2001	Immunogenicity of Therapeutic Biological Products
Vol. 113	Berlin, 2001	Process Validation for Manufacturing of Biologics and Biotechnology Products
Vol. 114	Ames, IA, 2002	Vaccines for OIE List A and Emerging Animal Diseases
Vol. 115	Bergen, 2002	Laboratory Correlates of Immunity to Influenza – A Reassessment,
Vol. 116	Los Angeles, CA, 2003	Development of Therapeutic Cancer Vaccines
Vol. 117	Langen, 2003	Consideration of Alternative Licensing Procedures for Vaccines for Minor Species, Minor Indications and Autogenous/Autologous Products
Vol. 118	Langen, 2003	PDA/EMEA European Virus Safety Forum
Vol. 119	Buenos Aires, 2004	Control of Infectious Animal Diseases by Vaccination
Vol. 120	Bethesda, MD, 2003	Advances in Transfusion Safety
Vol. 121	Bergen, 2003	Progress in Fish Vaccinology
Vol. 122	Bethesda, MD, 2003	State of the Art Analytical Methods for Characterization of Biological Products and Assessment of Comparability
Vol. 123	Rockville, MD, 2004	Vaccine Cell Substrates 2004
Vol. 124	Paris, France, 2005	OIE/FAO International Scientific Conference on Avian Influenza
Vol. 125	Kiev, Ukraine, 2005	First International Conference on Rabies in Europe
Vol. 126	Saint-Malo, France, 2005	New Diagnostic Technology: Applications in Animal Health and Biologics Controls
Vol. 127	Sydney, Australia, 2005	Advances in Transfusion Safety – Volume IV
Vol. 128	Florianopolis, Brazil, 2006	First International Conference of the OIE Reference Laboratories and Collaborating Centres